DID

- •IBS pain can mimic the symptoms of a heart attack.

- Many physicians prescribe unnecessary drugs.

- Female patients outnumber men two-to-one.

- Forty million Americans use laxatives every year—many in an attempt to ease the symptoms of IBS.

- Children and adolescents frequently suffer IBS symptoms they are too embarrassed to tell their parents about.

Information is your best weapon against IBS. For most people treatment is simple, inexpensive, and completely effective. You'll find everything you need to know in . . .

LEARNING TO LIVE WITH CHRONIC IBS

THE DELL MEDICAL LIBRARY

QUANTITY SALES

Most Dell books are available at special quantity discounts when purchased in bulk by corporations, organizations, and special-interest groups. Custom imprinting or excerpting can also be done to fit special needs. For details write: Dell Publishing, 666 Fifth Avenue, New York, NY 10103. Attn.: Special Sales Dept.

INDIVIDUAL SALES

Are there any Dell books you want but cannot find in your local stores? If so, you can order them directly from us. You can get any Dell book in print. Simply include the book's title, author, and ISBN number if you have it, along with a check or money order (no cash can be accepted) for the full retail price plus $2.00 to cover shipping and handling. Mail to: Dell Readers Service, P.O. Box 5057, Des Plaines, IL 60017.

Learning to Live with

CHRONIC IBS

Norra Tannenhaus

Foreword by Stephen M. Collins, M.D.

A LYNN SONBERG BOOK

Published by
Dell Publishing
a division of
Bantam Doubleday Dell Publishing Group, Inc.
666 Fifth Avenue
New York, New York 10103

Medical research about irritable bowel syndrome is ongoing and subject to interpretation. Although every effort has been made to include the most up-to-date and accurate information in this book, there can be no guarantee that what we know about IBS today won't change with time. Furthermore, IBS sometimes displays symptoms that may appear to be related to other ailments. The reader should bear in mind that this book is not for the purpose of self-diagnosis or self-treatment; he or she should consult appropriate medical professionals regarding all medical problems and any major dietary changes.

ISBN: 0-440-20597-2

Printed in the United States of America
Published simultaneously in Canada

June 1990

10 9 8 7 6 5 4 3 2 1

OPM

CONTENTS

ACKNOWLEDGMENTS

The author gratefully acknowledges the generosity and cooperation of Dr. Stephen M. Collins, Associate Professor of Medicine and Director, Intestinal Disease Research Unit, McMaster University Health Sciences Center, Hamilton, Ontario; Dr. Nathaniel Cohen, Associate Clinical Professor of Medicine and Chief, Gastroenterology Clinic, Mount Sinai Medical School, New York City; and Dr. Douglas A. Drossman, Associate Professor of Medicine and Psychiatry, Division of Digestive Diseases, University of North Carolina School of Medicine, Chapel Hill, North Carolina.

FOREWORD

This book's message is positive and optimistic: IBS is a benign, controllable disease. The author emphasizes a self-help approach that involves careful attention to symptoms, a patient approach to treatment, and a willingness to endure a little trial and error. With such an approach, the woman or man with IBS can minimize flare-ups or even, in many cases, send them into remission indefinitely.

Physicians' knowledge of IBS is increasing, and more attention is being paid to understanding the nature of bowel dysfunction, and thus the basis for symptoms. Although stress and behavioral factors influence the disease, IBS is *not* all in one's mind—it's also a functional disorder of the GI tract. Stress sometimes exacerbates IBS, but it may not necessarily cause the condition, and in many cases stress is not associated with flare-ups. In some patients, for example, IBS develops after an episode of infection in the bowel. We have much more to learn about the physiology of the GI tract before we can say with certainty why IBS occurs, but current evidence suggests that there may be a combination of factors, perhaps slightly different in each case, that initiates the disease and causes flare-ups. Until we know more about IBS and GI function, the best attitude is one of prudence. Effective treatment may be achieved through modification of diet and life-style, and, in some instances, with the help of drugs.

In this book Norra Tannenhaus explains what goes wrong in IBS and the different approaches to its treatment. She tells the reader how IBS is diagnosed, why doctors think it occurs, and, most important, how someone can regain control over his or her life. Through this book the reader will gain a clearer understanding of the nature of IBS and how it can be managed. Since the patient's attitude toward, and understanding of, his or her disease likely influences its prognosis, the information available through this book will help patients better manage their disease. The book is clearly written with the patient in mind.

IBS is one of the most common digestive disorders in the western world. Books such as this can help millions of sufferers learn more about their condition and, in so doing, immeasurably improve their lives.

Stephen M. Collins, M.D.
Director, Intestinal Disease Research Unit and
Associate Professor of Medicine,
McMaster University Health Sciences Center,
Ontario

INTRODUCTION

In our culture the digestive tract and its functions—and malfunctions—are often sources of humor, as well as some squeamishness. We would never discuss our bowel problems in polite society, and some people even feel embarrassed talking them over with a doctor. Yet, as the statistics below reveal, we're privately preoccupied with keeping our bowels clean and regular.

This year, forty million Americans will buy $225 million worth of laxatives. Of those forty million, twenty-four million—that's one out of every ten of us—will use those laxatives at least one to three times a month; roughly half of that group will regulate their bowels more than once a week.

Clearly digestive problems are extremely common. They cause more workplace absenteeism than the common cold and send more than five million people to the hospital every year. One out of every six major illnesses involves the digestive tract. As one expert put it, "Of all the systems in your body, your digestive system is most likely to give you trouble."

This book is about the commonest digestive disorder of all: irritable bowel syndrome, or IBS. No one knows exactly how many people have IBS because many sufferers do not discuss it. Some experts estimate that fifteen percent of the adult population has IBS; others claim the figure is closer to seventeen or nineteen percent. Others state their estimates in population figures, saying that while thirty million to forty million Americans have been diagnosed with IBS, as many as a hundred million people may have at least occasional episodes of it. In one study, one third of the subjects turned out to have symptoms of IBS.

Regardless of the figure you choose, one thing is clear: If you have IBS, you're not alone. It keeps a lot of doctors busy: up to seventy percent of all people referred by primary care physicians to gastroenterologists (doctors who specialize in the treatment of the digestive organs) are referred because they have symptoms of IBS, and these patients go on to form twenty-five percent of a given gastroenterologist's practice. One physician calls it "the common cold of the digestive tract."

IBS is a chronic disease, which means it is of long duration—persistence for at least two years is one diagnostic criterion. While it may strike anyone, its preferred targets appear to be people between the ages of twenty and fifty. Female patients outnumber males by about two to one.

The bad news about IBS is that there's no cure; once you've got it, you've got it. But there's also lots of good news about IBS. As unpleasant as its symptoms might be, it is *not* life threatening, and it does not damage any tissues or organs. It does not lead to more serious diseases. And, probably the best news of all: there is something you can do about it. IBS doesn't have to run your life; *you* can learn to control *it*. Many people become so skilled at managing their symptoms that their flare-ups virtually disappear. If and when an episode does occur, it is mild and short-lived. In fact, the successful control of IBS depends on the person who has it. Your history, symptoms, and triggering events may differ drastically from those of your mother, spouse, best friend, boss, or whoever else you know with this condition. It is, of course, essential to have your doctor's help as you learn how to control your IBS, but ultimately your doctor is only an educated guide and consultant—only *you* can determine what makes you feel better, and what makes you feel worse.

In this book you'll learn how you can manage your IBS, instead of allowing it to manage your life. The first half describes the symptoms of IBS, how and why doctors think it occurs, how it differs from other common digestive-tract conditions, and how it is diagnosed. Chapter One will explain what IBS is, why you have certain symptoms, and why symptoms vary among IBS sufferers. You'll learn something about the current state of knowledge regarding IBS, and why it is sometimes a challenge for doctors to diagnose. The questionnaire at the end of Chapter One is designed to help you determine if you have IBS; it may also help you do a little soul-searching as you think about what triggers your symptoms.

Chapter Two explains the interaction between your emotions and digestive-tract function. It describes a normally functioning digestive tract (also referred to as the gut), and it describes how the gut responds to stress. This information will then be tied together to show you how, and why, your gut may react—or overreact—to stressful situations, which are believed to be a major trigger of IBS.

How does your doctor diagnose IBS? That's the subject of Chapter Three, which describes the medical history, physical examination, and different kinds of tests doctors need to draw their conclusions. Chapter Three will also describe some other common disorders of the digestive tract, and how to distinguish them from IBS.

The second half of this book concentrates on the treatment of IBS and strategies for minimizing your symptoms and the situations that trigger them. It has one underlying idea: IBS treatment must be tailored to each patient, because each patient's experience with the disease is different from that of any other patient. Thus, you'll have to experiment with different therapies until you find something—or a combination of things—that works for you. Make your doctor your partner in therapy and devise a plan together that allows you to live comfortably with IBS.

Chapter Four discusses the effect of food on IBS. Along with presenting general information about diet that every IBS sufferer should know, this chapter explains why it's important to keep a food diary and how you can determine which foods trigger your symptoms. It also contains recommendations from the American Digestive Disease Society (ADDS).

To prescribe or not to prescribe drugs? This is one of the most controversial issues in the field of IBS therapy. Chapter Five takes a look at the drugs doctors most commonly prescribe for their patients with IBS, how these drugs work, and what their side effects may be. It will explain why some doctors think that prescription drugs are, for many patients, unnecessary. This chapter also discusses over-the-counter remedies IBS patients are most likely to use, most notably certain kinds of laxatives.

Chapter Six returns to the subject of stress. We'll review some of the findings about the relationship between IBS and an individual's response to stress, and why a daily diary is a good way to uncover stress-related triggers of your symptoms. In addition, safe and easy methods of coping with stress will be discussed, including biofeedback, relaxation techniques, and physical exercise.

Finally, Chapter Seven offers some general hints for living with IBS. Along with reviewing and summarizing the important points made elsewhere in the book, this chapter contains information on self-help programs for people with IBS, as well as other programs and coping methods for people with special problems. It closes with a list of organizations that can provide more information on many of the topics discussed in earlier chapters.

Remember: You don't have to be a prisoner of your symptoms. By reading this book, communicating with your doctor, making some changes in your life-style, and learning how to cope with stress, you can lead a normal, productive life with few—if any!—limitations. So turn the page and start living with IBS.

N.T.

PART I
UNDERSTANDING IBS

ONE

WHAT IS IBS?

"This has been happening ever since I was a child," said Margie, a newly promoted account executive at a major New York public-relations firm. "At the first sign of anything wrong, like a minor stomachache or if I ate breakfast too quickly and felt sick afterward, they would keep me home from school and put me to bed. Actually," she confessed with a sheepish smile, "it was sort of fun. I got to stay home, play with my toys and watch TV, and usually my father would bring me a little present when he came home from work.

"My IBS got worse after I entered adolescence and started getting my periods," she added, "but it's never been as bad as this. I find myself running to the bathroom six, seven, sometimes ten times a day. Sometimes the cramps are so bad, I can hardly walk. I was really afraid it would disrupt my wedding six months ago, but the worst embarrassment came last month, when my boss called me into her office to tell me I'd been promoted—I had to run out right after she gave me the good news!"

Sheila has a different story. "I had occasional flare-ups when I was a teenager, like the runs before a big exam, or cramps after a fight with my parents, but that didn't happen very often," she explained. "For the first few years after I got married, I didn't have any episodes at all because we were so happy together. Then my husband got a new job that required a lot of socializing—parties, dinners with clients, that sort of thing. I've really come to resent the time he spends away from his family, and the demands on me to accompany him to some of these gatherings. Now my stomach reminds me whenever I have to go a party with him—I'll start getting gas pains and diarrhea two days before."

Finally, there's Dave. "I've had a problem with gas and constipation for as long as I can remember, but I have no idea why. I've seen a doctor, and he said there's nothing wrong with me. I don't have any major problems in my life. I just try to live with it and take laxatives to keep myself regular." After reflecting for a moment he added, "My father had the same problem. I guess it runs in the family."

Does any of this sound familiar? Margie, Sheila, and Dave represent fairly typical cases of irritable bowel syndrome, or IBS. But even if your symptoms differ drastically, they may still be diagnosed as IBS. The fact is that each of the millions of people with IBS has a different story to tell.

IBS is a complex disorder that requires a sympathetic approach to treatment, although the treatment itself may be quite simple. IBS is a chronic disease, which means that it persists for a long time, usually years. You may go for extended periods without any problems, only to have a flare-up during a period of stress, after eating an unfamiliar food, or following a bout with a debilitating disease, like an intestinal virus. Or, as with Dave, your symptoms may occur for no apparent reason at all.

Whatever the cause, "living with IBS is no day at the beach," says one chronic sufferer. This is certainly true, but it need not be a perpetual purgatory either. The first step toward a fuller, more comfortable life with IBS is to learn more about this elusive and often frustrating condition.

THIS IS IBS

IBS is a challenging disease. Its symptoms vary from one patient to the next; doctors aren't certain what causes it; and, while many patients know what will trigger their symptoms, others claim there are no triggers at all—an episode may occur and subside spontaneously.

The confusion surrounding IBS is probably best reflected by the fact that IBS has many other names: spastic colon, spastic colon syndrome, irritable colon, colonic neurosis, nervous stomach, nervous diarrhea, functional bowel disease, mucous colitis, and chronic colitis. Actually, the last two names are inaccurate and have probably contributed to many misconceptions about IBS. IBS has nothing to do with colitis, an inflammatory disease that can be very serious. The differences between IBS and true colitis are discussed in Chapter Three.

SYMPTOMS OF IBS

The symptoms of IBS include:

—nausea
—gas
—heartburn

—diarrhea

—constipation

—alternating episodes of diarrhea and constipation

—gas pains extending to the lower back and sometimes even into the chest, neck, or down the left arm

—fatigue

—feelings of abdominal distension

—mucus in the stool

—the feeling that you haven't finished moving your bowels, a sensation doctors call "incomplete evacuation"

—occasionally, other health complaints such as headaches, colds, allergies, or pain in the back or joints

It's no wonder that so many IBS sufferers often feel tired, frustrated, and afraid of ever being too far from a bathroom. These symptoms fluctuate in severity and usually don't occur all at once, but in one study ninety-nine percent of the patients had at least two symptoms at a time.

Most patients experience one of three possible patterns of symptoms. In one, there is pain, gas distension, and the feeling of being bloated; constipation alternates with diarrhea.

The second pattern is characterized by frequent bouts of constipation, and in the third, patients report diarrhea as the primary symptom.

As you read this you may be thinking, "So what? Who hasn't had heartburn or diarrhea at least once in their lives?" This is true; virtually all of us have experienced symptoms like these at one time or another. The difference between someone with an occasional gas pain and someone else with full-blown IBS is one of number, frequency, and degree: the symptoms of the IBS patient are more numerous, and they are frequent and severe enough to disrupt the patient's life.

TWO IMPORTANT FACTS ABOUT IBS

As you learn more about this condition, keep two facts in mind. First, no matter how troublesome your symptoms, remember that *IBS is not associated with any serious complications and has no known link to colon cancer or any other life-threatening condition.* Its severity is determined primarily by the discomfort it causes you and the restrictions it places on your life.

Second, it's important to realize that although IBS itself is not a life-threatening condition, its symptoms sometimes mimic those of other, more serious diseases. In younger people they may approximate symptoms of Crohn's disease or ulcerative colitis, two common inflammatory diseases of the gut that can lead to permanent disability. With older patients doctors think of colon polyps or colon cancer.* Therefore, self-diagnosis is not a good idea. It's essential to let your doctor determine the exact nature of your condition.

WHO GETS IBS?

IBS is common in the United States, Japan, South America, India, and Sri Lanka, although for some reason it is rare in African countries such as Uganda. In the western

*These conditions are described more fully in Chapter Three.

world female patients outnumber male patients by two to one, but in India and Sri Lanka only twenty to thirty percent of all IBS patients are women—in other words, the male patients outnumber the females by a ratio of as much as five to one. Some experts think these numbers reflect not the true ratio of male versus female IBS sufferers, but health-care habits in different societies. In the United States women are more likely to visit doctors for any reason, while in India doctors are more often visited by men.

There's some evidence that IBS runs in families, so if your father or Aunt Tillie had IBS, the chances are greater that you will have it too. It's also been found that people who develop migraine headaches are at greater risk of developing IBS.

IBS sufferers are often in their twenties, thirties, or forties, with about half the patients seen before age thirty-five. Symptoms typically begin sometime during childhood or adolescence. In fact, the sudden onset of symptoms in an older person who has no history of IBS in childhood, adolescence, or early adulthood usually means that the condition is something other than IBS.

IT'S NOT IN YOUR HEAD

"My doctor did all sorts of tests, and he can't find anything wrong with me." If you suffer from IBS or know someone who does, these words probably sound familiar. In the past many doctors would pat the IBS patient on the back and say, "There's nothing wrong with you—it's all in your head." Today, most physicians realize that while their tests may not reveal anything out of the ordinary, your symptoms are still very real. Thus, they describe IBS as a *functional bowel disorder*. This means there is a disorder in the functioning of the gut for which doctors can find no apparent structural or biochemical cause with the technology available to them right now. Some experts think it may be possible to detect the precise cause of the malfunction someday. Currently, however, the most that can be said is that in some people, the intestine is simply more sensitive to certain environmental factors such as food or stress.

As you'll see in Chapter Two, the digestive tract relaxes and contracts in a characteristic way, so it can push the food along and digest it properly. The symptoms of IBS result when this rhythm is disturbed. When the digestive tract contracts too slowly, constipation results; when it contracts too rapidly or goes into spasm, diarrhea occurs. This irregular propulsive action also leads to the trapping of gas.

These two problems, the abnormal contractions of the tract, and the gas trapped by these disordered movements, are what cause the pain of IBS. Gas trapped on the left side of the colon can lead to pain that radiates to the chest and down the left shoulder or arm, creating symptoms similar to those of a heart attack. Pain in other parts of the colon may radiate to the back, imitating serious disorders like kidney stones, gallbladder disease, or appendicitis. If it's IBS that's causing the pain, however, relief should come by expelling the gas or moving your bowels. *Nevertheless, don't self-diagnose: if your pain is severe and recurs frequently, see your doctor for a thorough checkup and an accurate diagnosis. If the pain is in your chest, left shoulder, or left arm, don't wait—call your doctor immediately.* Better safe than sorry.

WHAT CAUSES IBS?

Perhaps it's now a bit clearer why doctors are still baffled by IBS. Until they can discover what causes the functional problems, they won't be able to determine exactly what causes IBS or why some people get it and some don't. With the information that's currently available, most experts say that some people are simply more prone to IBS, the way others are more prone to backaches, asthma, or migraine headaches. (One physician describes IBS as "the asthma of the gut.") Like IBS these are all real physiological conditions in which different triggering events, such as stress, interact with each person's unique "chemistry" (used here in a figurative, not a literal, sense) to create a flare-up.

Because of this interaction among physiology, personal traits, and outside triggering occurrences, doctors describe IBS as a biopsychosocial disorder. Indeed, IBS is only one of many conditions in which biological factors combine with psychological characteristics and social pressures to initiate an episode of that condition, or to make symptoms worse once they've begun.

Many things can trigger an episode of IBS. Some people trace its development to a particularly severe viral infection, like a bout with an intestinal bug or the flu. Others find their symptoms triggered by certain medicines, like antibiotics or narcotics. There are, however, three major culprits: diet, hormones, and stress. Each of these factors is covered in more detail later in the book, but as you read about them remember that none of them exists in a vacuum. Sheila, for example, loves eggs and usually eats them with no problem, but a few days before one of her husband's work-related parties, they'll send her running to the bathroom. Margie, the newly promoted account executive, thrives on her work, but if she works late while she's having her period, her stomach makes her sorry. Even Dave, after a little introspection, found that his episodes of constipation usually seemed to occur right around the Christmas holidays, which always leave him happy but exhausted from entertaining family and friends.

In short, troublesome items or events interact with one another to trigger your episodes of IBS. A food you usually eat with impunity may become your worst enemy when you're tired or under stress. Perhaps you love your high-pressure job, but your new boss reminds you of your mother-in-law and you no longer bother to put away your bathroom key. If you're a woman, your IBS may be particularly bad at certain times of the month, when hormonal changes combine with the other events in your life to turn your bowels to water. On the other hand, you may associate your IBS with that bug you picked up during a trip to Mexico or the medicine your dentist gave you for an abscessed tooth. If you keep these examples in mind, you may find it easier to determine what triggers your symptoms as you learn to live with IBS.

QUESTIONNAIRE:
DO YOU HAVE IBS?

The questions that follow were designed to help you think about your symptoms in more detail. Through such introspection, you may be able to recognize certain symptom patterns or particular circumstances under which they flare. This will give you more insight into your condition and will allow you to answer your doctor's questions more precisely. There are no "right" or "wrong" answers.

Do not use this questionnaire for self-diagnosis! Only your doctor can determine what you really have. Instead, think of these questions as one of the tools that can help you improve your life—under your doctor's guidance.

I. Your Symptoms and the Circumstances Under Which They Occur

1. Which of the following do you experience on a regular or predictable basis? (Check as many as apply to you.)

   —constipation

   —diarrhea

   —gas

   —abdominal cramps

   —gas pains

   —unexplained pain in the chest, arm, or shoulder

   —nausea

   —heartburn

   —burping

   —the feeling that you're bloated or your stomach is distended

   —the feeling that you haven't moved your bowels completely

The symptoms of IBS are described as "nonspecific," because they may indicate one of any number of condi-

tions. The items listed above are, however, the symptoms most commonly associated with IBS.

2. How long have these symptoms occurred and recurred? (Check one.)

—Ever since I was a child or teenager
—For the past five years or more
—For the past two to five years
—For less than one year

IBS is a chronic, or long-lasting, condition. Many doctors use two years or more as a rough guide for a diagnosis of IBS.

3. Which of the following statements best applies to you? (There may be more than one.)

—I'll be fine for weeks or months and then suddenly, without warning, my symptoms will recur.
—I've got it down to a science: I know I'll be sorry if I eat certain food, talk to certain people, push myself too hard, or place myself in certain situations.
—My symptoms are unpredictable. Something that triggers them on one occasion may be perfectly benign on another.

For premenopausal women only: To avoid flare-ups, I've got to be careful at certain times of the month.

Any of these symptom patterns may be characteristic of IBS. What is not characteristic is pain or bowel problems that persist no matter what you do. This signals the presence of something other than IBS, and indicates that a trip to the doctor is in order.

4. Do any of the following foods disagree with you?

—coffee or tea

—chocolate

—beans, cabbage, or other gas-producing foods

—whole-grain breads or cereals or other high-fiber foods

—artificial sweeteners

—milk and milk products

Any or all of these may trigger flare-ups in the person with IBS.

5. Do you frequently experience any of these?

—headaches

—backaches

—frequent colds, "sniffles," or the flu

—joint pain

Some people with IBS have these conditions as well.

6. Are you ever awakened by abdominal pain?

This is definitely not a symptom of IBS, but it may indicate another common gut disorder such as ulcerative colitis or Crohn's disease.

II. Recent Stress in Your Life

7. How many of the following stressful events have you experienced within the past two years?

—death of a spouse

—divorce

—marital separation

—a jail term
—death of a close family member
—personal illness or injury
—marriage
—fired at work
—marital reconciliation
—retirement
—change in health of a family member
—pregnancy
—sexual difficulties
—gain of a new family member
—change in financial status
—death of a close friend
—change to a different line of work
—change in the number of arguments with your spouse
—foreclosure of a mortgage or a loan
—change in responsibilities at work
—son or daughter leaving home
—trouble with in-laws
—outstanding personal achievement
—spouse begins or stops work
—begin or end school
—trouble with your boss
—change in residence
—change in schools
—change in sleeping habits
—change in eating habits
—vacation
—Christmas
—minor violations of the law

These are considered (in descending order of importance) the major forms of stress in a person's life. If your IBS symptoms are triggered by stress, any of these events may spell danger for you.

8. How do you handle stress when it arises? (Check as many as apply to you.)

—I engage in some physical exercise.

—I talk to my psychotherapist, minister, counselor, or close friend.

—I work on a hobby.

—I take a vacation.

—I go out for a night on the town.

—I buy myself a little present.

—I read, watch TV, or go to a movie or a play.

—I engage in some relaxation exercise such as meditation.

—I try to ignore stress as best I can and not let it interfere with my life.

—Who has stress? My life is very calm.

The first eight items are constructive ways of handling stress. The two final items indicate that you bottle up your stressful feelings by ignoring them or denying them completely. Your bowel, however, may feel the consequence.

TWO

GUT FEELINGS

When something afflicts an organ as complex as the gut,* it is highly unlikely that one specific abnormality is the cause. What's more probable is that several malfunctioning mechanisms interact in a given patient, with the precise combination of malfunctions differing from one person to the next.

An episode of IBS may be triggered by many things, but one of the primary instigators is stress. Chapter Six looks at the ambiguous and highly subjective concept of stress in detail, but what's important to know now is that "stress"—however you define it, however you perceive it—can have a profound effect upon body systems, and the digestive system is one of its favorite targets. The explosion of stress research that's occurred since the end of World War II has yielded some fascinating information about the connection between the body and the mind. Some of this research has emphasized the effects of stress on the digestive system, and particularly the differences in stress response between people with IBS and those without it.

---

*Throughout this book the terms *gut, digestive tract, digestive system, gastrointestinal tract,* and *GI tract* will be used interchangeably.

In this chapter we'll look at some of the ways in which digestive-tract function goes awry when you have IBS. But we cannot begin to explain how and why the digestive system fails without first explaining how the system works when it is healthy and functioning properly, so let's first take a brief look at the normal function of the GI tract.

THE HEALTHY DIGESTIVE SYSTEM

Think of your body as a doughnut, with your digestive tract as the hole. Everything you pour down that hole remains outside the body, until the digestive tract breaks it down into a form suitable for absorption and use by the cells. This, then, is the purpose of digestion: to break down everything you eat and drink into smaller, simpler nutrient molecules, which can then cross from the walls of the digestive tract into your blood or lymph and travel to the various organs.

The digestive tract—also called the gastrointestinal, or GI, tract—uses two basic tools for digesting food. One is movement. Your GI tract is built partly of muscles that relax and contract to mix the food thoroughly and move it along as it's worked upon by the other tool, which we'll call the "intestinal juices." This term refers to the array of hormones, enzymes, and other substances the gut uses to break the food down. These intestinal juices may come from specialized areas in the gut itself, or they may arise from the glands and organs that work in conjunction with the gut: the liver, pancreas, and gallbladder.

DIGESTION

Digestion begins in the mouth. By chewing your food and mixing it with saliva, you prepare it for being swallowed and reduced into an absorbable form. Saliva moistens the food and contains enzymes which start the breakdown process.

Muscular contractions propel swallowed food through the throat (doctors call this organ the pharynx) into the esophagus, which stretches from the chest to the stomach. Imagine a piece of food traveling through the throat and esophagus as a piece of food traveling through a snake; as the food reaches a certain area of the snake's body, the muscles in that area contract to push the food down. So it is with the GI tract, with muscles in the esophagus alternately contracting and relaxing to let the food travel to the stomach.

The stomach acts as a mixing or churning vat. Stomach cells release enzymes and hydrochloric acid, which further break down the food. Stomach cells also release fluid that mixes with the food as it's being digested. While this is going on, stomach movements churn the mass of food, acid, and stomach juices to ensure adequate mixing. The result is a semiliquid substance that's ready to proceed down the digestive tract to the small intestine.

Once the food reaches the small intestine, digestion continues and absorption begins. Cells of the small intestine release fluid that adjust the chemical composition of the digested mass, so that it's in a form suitable for further breakdown and absorption. At the same time other cells release hormones that, in turn, signal the liver, gallbladder, and pancreas to release their digestive juices and continue the breakdown of the food. One of these hormones, cholecystokinin, or CCK, is thought to influence the symptoms of IBS. This will be explained in more detail later in the chapter.

Once the intestinal actions and juices break down the food into its simplest components, these components are absorbed from the walls of the small intestine into the blood and lymph. Vitamins, minerals, and any drugs you might have taken are absorbed from the small intestine as well.

From the small intestine what's left of your meal enters the colon (large intestine). If your GI tract is working properly, all of the nutrients—vitamins, minerals, fats, carbohydrates, and protein—will have been absorbed into the body by this point. The waste that remains consists mainly of water, some dissolved salts and bodily secretions, and indigestible material such as fiber.

Some experts describe the colon as a "drying vat." That's because its main job is to absorb water and salt from the material that enters from the small intestine. The colon can absorb more than two quarts of liquid a day; with more fluid than that, an excessively watery stool may result—diarrhea.

The colon moves slowly, especially when compared to the small intestine. The muscles of the large intestine require several minutes to contract and relax, while in the small intestine, the same thing happens in a matter of seconds. After a meal the colon's contents travel forward at about 4.4 inches per hour, although certain drugs can speed this to 8 inches per hour. Between meals the colon's movements subside, and whatever material it contains travels at roughly 2 inches per hour. In people who are constipated, colonic contents may move less than half an inch per hour. Dr. Horace Davenport, the author of a classic medical textbook on digestion, once wrote, "Slow and reluctant is the long descent with many a lingering farewell look behind."

WHAT GOES WRONG IN IBS?

IBS is essentially a disorder of motility: the muscles of the digestive tract do not contract properly, so that the movement of food is excessively fast or slow. Most discussions of IBS emphasize the colon, or large intestine, but actually this condition may involve any portion of the digestive tract. Some IBS patients report symptoms that suggest delayed emptying of stomach contents into the small intestine:

—Feelings of being bloated
—A persistent feeling of being uncomfortably full
—Stomach discomfort or heartburn
—Nausea and possible vomiting

In addition, some investigators have detected irregular activity in the muscles of the esophagus and small intestine of IBS patients, both spontaneously and under experimental conditions.

More recent research has been able to identify some abnormal patterns of activity in the colons of people with IBS. In some cases they can correlate symptoms with this abnormal activity.

Movements of the colon are controlled by nerves and hormones and by electrical activity in the colon muscle. The electrical activity serves as a "pacemaker" similar to the mechanism that controls heart function. In people who have IBS, the muscle of the lower portion of the colon contracts abnormally. An abnormal contraction, or spasm, may be related to episodes of crampy pain. Sometimes the spasm delays the passage of stool, leading to constipation. At other times the spasm leads to more rapid passage of feces and the result is diarrhea.

Here again, painful spasms are not limited to the colon. In some people abdominal pain has been correlated with spasms in the small intestine.

THE ROLE OF CCK

Earlier in this chapter you read about one of the gut hormones, cholecystokinin, also called CCK. Released in response to food entering the small intestine, CCK stimulates contractions of the intestinal tract to keep food moving along, and it also acts on the gallbladder to aid indirectly in the digestion of fatty foods. In people with IBS, CCK may overstimulate the colon, causing it to contract too rapidly and rush the waste through, resulting in diarrhea. If you get diarrhea after eating a rich, heavy meal, this could be the reason.

AN OVERSENSITIVE GUT?

Today most experts believe that IBS patients have a "hyperactive gut": that is, their GI tracts overreact to agents that stimulate a normal gut in a more moderate fashion. Some of these agents include:

—certain kinds of drugs
—CCK
—meals or certain kinds of food
—experimental distension of the rectum
—psychological stress

It follows that, because an IBS patient's gut is unduly sensitive to such stimuli, he or she will feel worse than a non-IBS sufferer when exposed to these items. In stressful situations, for example, recent studies indicate that the GI tracts of IBS patients are more likely than others to overreact to anger, sadness, or anxiety.

STRESS AND THE GUT

It's well known that stress can affect the function of the GI tract. In a classic series of experiments conducted in the nineteen forties, Dr. Thomas Almy and his colleagues demonstrated that, when exposed to situations that provoked anger, colon pressure in healthy subjects and in people with IBS went up, and constipation resulted. Under conditions of sadness and anxiety, colon pressure went down, and diarrhea occurred. When the experimenters elicited feelings of tension and fear by telling the subjects that they might have rectal cancer, colon pressure went up and stayed up until the people were given a clean bill of health.

It is also known that gut hormones such as CCK are also made in the brain, creating a "gut-brain axis" through which these two organs can communicate with each other, allowing for the precise regulation of digestive-tract function: the contraction of muscles, opening and closing of valves, and secretion of digestive juices from glands and specialized cells. Thus, chronic stress and other behavioral factors may affect GI function, and signals from an unusually sensitive GI tract may be transmitted to the brain. Add to this an individual's personality traits and idiosyncrasies, and the result is a syndrome that varies from one patient to the next.

THE MAJOR SYMPTOMS OF IBS

The problems in motility seen in IBS lead directly to two of its most common and troublesome symptoms: constipation and diarrhea.

Constipation

Many people believe that good health includes a bowel movement every day. They worry when one or two days go by without a movement and panic when the days number three or more. But in fact, "regularity" is a highly individual thing: some people defecate after every meal, while others go only once every three days and feel fine. So how do you know if you're constipated?

Constipation is probably best defined as a hard bowel movement passed with discomfort, difficulty, or pain. You may have to strain on the toilet to evacuate completely. The stools are dry and hard because they've remained in the colon too long and have had too much water taken out.

Doctors today discourage their patients from thinking of constipation in terms of time elapsed between bowel movements. As a general rule, if several days pass but movements occur without discomfort, you're probably not constipated. But for people who feel reassured by numbers, most experts believe that at least three days must elapse before they will consider a diagnosis of constipation. Other symptoms of constipation include:

—restlessness

—dull headache

—depression

—loss of appetite, sometimes accompanied by nausea

—bad breath

—coated tongue

—abdominal distension

Pain, or the anticipation of pain, can inhibit the urge to defecate, and depression is known to cause constipation. So it's not hard to see how constipation, whether or not it's part of the larger picture of IBS, can result during periods of stress.

Diarrhea

At the other end of the spectrum lies diarrhea, probably best described as a condition characterized by loose, watery stools accompanied by a sense of urgency. Here again, physicians warn against paying too much attention to the frequency of bowel movements.

Just as constipation results when colon motility is too slow, diarrhea occurs when it is too fast, and intestinal contents rush through before enough water has been absorbed. And, as with constipation, diarrhea may be stress related. Many a college student has had a bout with the runs the night before a final exam!

If your diarrhea is associated with IBS, the first bowel movement of the day will probably consist of loose, semiformed stools, with subsequent stools containing less and less fecal matter and more and more mucus. The mucus, which resembles raw egg white, reflects the abnormal colon motility that is part of IBS and does *not* indicate the presence of a more serious condition, like inflammation or infection.

GUT FEELINGS: CONCLUSION

GI tract function is regulated by a variety of nerves, muscles, hormones, and "juices." That this complex system works so well so often is one of the miracles of biology. But it is this very complexity that makes the GI tract so vulnerable to malfunction.

Today most experts think the symptoms of IBS result from GI-tract motility problems associated with the gut's tendency to overreact to factors such as food, hormones, and stress. Stress, in particular, has a clear influence on the function of the GI tract, and IBS is closely associated with episodes of stress.

These changes in motility lead to the two major symptoms associated with IBS: constipation and diarrhea. Constipation results when intestinal motility is too slow; diarrhea results when it is too fast. These conditions can be treated, but can make one's life miserable nevertheless.

Constipation and diarrhea are not, however, unique to IBS; they may be associated with a number of other conditions. In fact, none of the symptoms of IBS is unique to IBS alone. How do you know your symptoms indicate IBS and not something else? Only your doctor can tell you for sure, as described in Chapter Three.

THREE

IS IT REALLY IBS?

IBS is a functional disorder, so even when you feel miserable, diagnostic tests reveal nothing amiss. Therefore, doctors must diagnose IBS based on what their tests and findings do *not* show, along with the information you give them. This is called a diagnosis of exclusion because the doctor excludes other possibilities to arrive at a diagnosis of IBS.

FINDING THE RIGHT PHYSICIAN

Communication between patient and physician is always important, but it's critical when you have a condition as disruptive and embarrassing as IBS. Therefore it's important to find a doctor you like and can trust.

Specialist or General Practitioner?

General practitioners, also called family practitioners or GPs, treat most common complaints that do not require specialized training or equipment. Sometimes people use a specialist in one area as their GP for everything; for example, many women look to their gynecologists as their general practitioners. If you have a GP with whom you're comfortable and who keeps your IBS under control, by all means stay with that doctor.

But what happens if your symptoms confound your family doctor or if they become more severe? Then it's probably time to visit a specialist, a doctor who limits his or her practice to the treatment of one class of diseases or one organ or organ system. As an IBS patient you'd most likely need a specialist known as a gastroenterologist, who confines his or her practice to the treatment of diseases of the gut.

What to Look for in a Physician

Ideally, you should shop for a doctor as carefully as you'd shop for a refrigerator or a car. Unfortunately, most of us don't bother to look for a doctor until we're sick and don't have time to shop around, and all too often we allow ourselves to be more impressed by degrees and diplomas than by personality or that quality known as "bedside manner." Of course it's important that your doctor be competent, but it's also essential that you can talk freely with him. If you can't be honest with your doctor and tell him everything, he won't be able to help you. For people who don't yet have a physician or are thinking of finding a new one, here are a few qualities to keep in mind:

—He answers questions quickly and clearly; he respects your feelings and allows you to express your fears about your symptoms or certain forms of treatment.

—He is knowledgeable about preventive measures that will help you avoid IBS attacks, instead of just treating them as they occur.

—He explains any medical tests or procedures before he performs them and warns you of any pain or discomfort, or of possible side effects of drugs prescribed.

—He takes your symptoms seriously and doesn't try to convince you that there's nothing wrong with you.

—He treats you courteously and sees you promptly.

—If you're seeing a general practitioner, he recognizes the limits of the care he can provide and will refer you to a specialist when necessary.

—If you're seeing a gastroenterologist, he has experience treating people with IBS (typically IBS patients may form twenty-five percent or more of a gastroenterologist's practice), and is a fellow of the American College of Gastroenterologists, which certifies that a physician is qualified to specialize in this area.

To make a diagnosis of IBS or any other condition, a physician relies upon three basic tools: the medical history you provide, your physical examination, and tests such as X rays and blood tests when the symptoms warrant them. People with IBS used to endure an extensive battery of costly, uncomfortable, and potentially dangerous tests, so their doctors could rule out every other possible diagnosis. Today, however, such exhaustive investigations are discouraged in the belief that IBS can be accurately diagnosed using the approach described above. This method has a good track record: according to a recent study, it leads to an accurate diagnosis ninety-five to ninety-eight percent of the time.

THE MEDICAL HISTORY

Many experts believe that a thorough medical history is the most important component in the diagnosis of IBS. A medical history is simply a record of your symptoms and any past illnesses or other health problems you've had. But this simple definition belies the history's importance: through the right questions an astute physician can ferret out information critical to an accurate diagnosis. That's why a certain amount of soul searching, like that encouraged by the questionnaire in Chapter One, may be helpful. Some questions you may expect from your doctor are:

—What is your problem?

—When did your symptoms begin?

—What seems to trigger your symptoms?

—Do you associate any major life events with the onset of your symptoms?

—Have you experienced any recent stress?

—What form of treatment have you tried in the past? How did it work?

—Why are you seeking help now?

—Are you looking for a cure?

—Have you recently run a fever or lost weight without trying?

You can help your doctor by supplying this information:

—What do you mean when you say you're constipated? Some people feel constipated if they don't move their bowels for two days; others don't worry until a week has passed.

—A description of your use of laxatives and any other drugs, prescription or over-the-counter, even if you don't think it has anything to do with your symptoms.

If your doctor doesn't ask, offer this information:

—Recent stresses you've undergone.
—When your symptoms began and what seems to trigger them.
—The treatment you've already tried and how it has worked.
—Any recent change in bowel frequency or in the consistency or color, or the appearance of blood in the stool.
—Any episode of pain that has disrupted your sleep.

THE PHYSICAL EXAMINATION

After taking your medical history the doctor will give you a physical examination. Most physicians take into account the patient's age, symptoms, medical history, and general health when they conduct the exam. Specialty also makes a difference: a general practitioner will examine you differently than a gastroenterologist. In general, however, during the exam you can probably expect your doctor to do the following:

—Listen to your heart and lungs, using the stethoscope
—Listen for characteristic bowel sounds with the stethoscope on your abdomen
—Check your blood pressure
—Check your reflexes
—Examine your eyes with an ophthalmoscope

—Administer a rectal examination by inserting a finger into your rectum, particularly if you're constipated

—Feel your abdomen for tenderness or abdominal masses

Some unexpected things your doctor may do:

—Look at your neck for signs of an overactive thyroid, which may cause diarrhea

—Look at your lips and in your mouth. Freckled lips sometimes indicate the presence of colon polyps (discussed in more detail below), while tiny red spots on the lips, tongue, or lining of the mouth suggest the presence of dilated blood vessels, which may also be in the stomach or intestine and cause GI bleeding.

—Administer a neurological examination to rule out problems such as diabetic neuropathy, which may cause intestinal symptoms

If your exam reveals no other problems, and assuming your history is typical of that for someone with IBS, your doctor will probably diagnose IBS. However, depending on your age, the severity and duration of your symptoms, and the results of your physical exam, he may decide to perform certain diagnostic tests.

COMMON DIAGNOSTIC TESTS

The diagnostic tests most commonly performed on people with bowel disorders include:

—Blood tests for anemia. The presence of anemia suggests the possibility that blood from the colon is oozing into the stool.

—Stool analyses for parasites, which may be the cause of your symptoms, or for blood, for further evidence of gastrointestinal bleeding.

If the tests do reveal signs of bleeding, your doctor will probably order X rays and/or a colonoscopy.

X Rays

X rays provide doctors with a picture of an organ, in this case the GI tract, and any physical abnormalities it may contain. There are two ways to X ray the GI tract: with an upper GI series, or with a barium enema X ray. As its name implies, the upper GI series X rays the upper GI tract, primarily the stomach and small intestine. For this test the patient drinks a special solution that makes the upper GI tract, including any abnormalities that might be present, visible on X ray film.

The barium enema X ray is used if the doctor suspects an abnormality in the lower GI tract, including the colon and rectum. Here again a special solution makes the organ visible on X ray film, but this time the solution, called barium, is administered by enema. Hence the name, barium enema X ray.

Colonoscopy and Sigmoidoscopy

The purpose of the colonoscope and sigmoidoscope is to offer doctors a direct view into the colon, to let them photograph the colon's interior, and to permit them to gather tissue samples (biopsies) that they can examine under a microscope. In some cases they may even be able to reproduce some of the patient's symptoms, so they can get a firsthand look at the colon's response to certain stimuli.

A colonoscope is basically a long, hollow tube with a light attached at one end. By feeding this tube, lit end first, into the anus and rectum and up into the colon, the doctor can see virtually the entire length of that organ. The sigmoidoscope is a newer form of colonoscope, and is shorter to permit observation of only the lower ten- to fifteen-inch portion of the colon, known as the sigmoid colon.

Colonoscopy is probably one of the least dignified medical tests in existence. A day or two before the test you'll receive laxatives or enemas to clean out your colon, and you'll probably be instructed to drink only clear liquids during this time to keep the colon clean. If more rapid cleansing is required you may have to drink one or two quarts of salt water just before the exam. People with high blood pressure cannot tolerate this much salt, so if you have this condition, tell your doctor.

On the day of the exam you'll receive a sedative. This will relax you and help relieve the physical discomfort you may feel while the tube is being inserted. Most patients feel less uncomfortable with the sigmoidoscope, which is shorter and more flexible and moves more easily through the colon. In fact, some physicians include sigmoidoscopy in their first battery of tests, and go on to the colonoscope only if they find any evidence of blood.

WHAT ELSE COULD IT BE?

The symptoms of IBS do indeed appear in many other conditions, but there are usually other symptoms or signs that distinguish these conditions from IBS. One general rule of thumb is that most serious digestive diseases will eventually cause a loss of weight even if the patient isn't dieting. IBS, on the other hand, does not usually lead to weight loss.

Still, there is a long list of conditions whose symptoms may mimic those of IBS. The ones doctors most commonly suspect are:

—diverticulosis
—diverticulitis
—Crohn's disease
—ulcerative colitis
—colon cancer
—colon polyps

Let's look at each one in turn.

Diverticulosis and Diverticulitis

Many ailments have been attributed to modern civilization, and diverticulosis is one of them. This condition, in which pouches, or diverticuli, develop in the lining of the colon and eventually protrude from that organ, is thought to result from the fiber-poor diets and stress-filled lives we lead today. Diverticulitis sets in when those pouches become irritated and inflamed.

The symptoms of diverticulosis vary, but usually they include abdominal cramps after you eat foods like nuts, popcorn, and items containing seeds, all of which contain a certain kind of fiber that irritates the diverticuli. Abdominal pain is also a symptom of diverticulitis, only this pain is more severe and is associated with fever and sometimes chills. The pain is often concentrated around the lower left part of the abdomen, and may intensify with walking or any other form of movement.

Some doctors think IBS may sometimes herald the development of diverticulosis. Diverticuli probably result when gas or stool become trapped in the colon and create pockets of high pressure, from which diverticuli then form. Since trapped gas and constipation are symptoms of IBS, these conditions may be somehow linked.

Crohn's Disease

One of the most serious digestive-tract diseases, Crohn's disease (named for the physician who studied it extensively, but also called regional ileitis) is a chronic inflammation of the digestive tract. This inflammation leads to ulceration of the gut lining, through which the patient may lose blood, fluids, and protein, ultimately leading to anemia, dehydration, or malnutrition. The ulcerated areas may thicken and form scars that sometimes block the GI tract and cause intestinal obstruction. Crohn's disease may affect any portion of the GI tract, but it occurs most often in the colon.

When the outer layers of the intestine become severely inflamed, they may form an abnormal connection with another organ, such as the bladder, one of the female sex organs, other parts of the digestive system, or even the skin. These connections, known as fistulas, are responsible for many of the symptoms and complications of Crohn's disease. The symptoms vary with the part of the digestive tract involved, but Crohn's disease of the colon is characterized by bloody diarrhea, weight loss, and possible malnutrition. Symptoms of Crohn's disease of the small intestine include:

—diarrhea, with or without blood
—frequent loose bowel movements associated with abdominal cramps
—anemia
—weight loss
—malnutrition, including possible vitamin deficiencies if the small intestine cannot absorb nutrients
—malaise, fatigue

People who develop intestinal obstructions due to scarring may experience:

—severe cramps and stomach pain
—vomiting after eating solid food

Like IBS, Crohn's disease may go into remission for a while only to flare up periodically.

Currently there is no cure for Crohn's disease. When possible, patients are offered relief for their symptoms. Sometimes doctors will surgically remove a severely damaged portion of the intestinal tract, only to have the Crohn's disease recur in some other area.

Ulcerative Colitis

Like Crohn's disease, ulcerative colitis consists of chronic inflammation and ulceration of the gut lining, marked by flare-ups and periods of remission. Its cause is unknown.

Unlike Crohn's disease, ulcerative colitis is localized to one portion of the GI tract: the colon.

The symptoms of ulcerative colitis include cramps, weight loss, rectal bleeding after a bowel movement, and diarrhea that may become urgent—patients have been known to have accidents. Many people awaken several times during the night to go to the bathroom, and someone in the throes of a full-fledged attack may run to the john up to twenty times a day. These episodes are often associated with fatigue, fever, weakness, loss of appetite, and loss of weight.

Ulcerative colitis differs from Crohn's disease in one other respect: it is curable, through surgical removal of the colon.

Inflammatory Bowel Diseases vs. IBS

Because they are both characterized by inflammation and share certain symptoms, Crohn's disease and ulcerative colitis are often referred to together as the inflammatory bowel diseases. IBS differs from these diseases in some important ways:

—IBS is *not* associated with any form of inflammation. This is why names for IBS that include the word *colitis*, which implies the presence of inflammation, are inaccurate and confusing.

—The diarrhea associated with IBS rarely occurs after you fall asleep, and it never contains blood.

—IBS does not involve fever, weight loss, anemia, or malnutrition.

—People with inflammatory bowel diseases run a higher-than-average risk of developing cancer of the colon or rectum; people with IBS do not.

Colon Cancer and Colon Polyps

Colon cancer is one of the commonest forms of cancer in the United States, and is thought to be related to the high-fat, low-fiber diet so many of us consume. However, if caught and treated in time, colon cancer is highly curable and its patients can lead a full and normal life.

Colon cancer originates in the lining of the colon and, as it grows, protrudes into the colon cavity through which the feces pass. If allowed to grow large enough, a colon tumor can obstruct fecal movement.

The symptoms of colon cancer may vary, depending upon the part of the colon in which the tumor is found. In general, blood in the stool is a sign of early colon cancer. Other possible symptoms and signs are:

—Rectal bleeding resembling the bleeding seen with hemorrhoids, for which this is sometimes misdiagnosed

—Abdominal cramps that may be partially relieved by a bowel movement

—Dull, persistent abdominal pain

—Rectal pain

—Persistent constipation or diarrhea

—Alternating constipation and diarrhea

—General weakness or fatigue if there is heavy loss of blood

—A change in bowel habits, including:
  difficulty in moving one's bowels
  a feeling of fullness in the rectum, or a feeling as though you have to move your bowels but are unable to do so

a narrowing of stool diameter, leading to stools sometimes described as "pencillike"

—Loss of appetite or weight

Colon cancer is often diagnosed from a rectal examination. If the doctor needs more information he'll probably
perform a colonoscopy, using a form of that instrument
called a proctosigmoidoscope. Because early colon cancer
can be so easily detected from a rectal exam, the American Cancer Society recommends this procedure annually
for everyone over the age of forty.

Currently the best treatment for colon cancer is surgical removal of the tumor and any lymph nodes to which
it may have spread.

Colon polyps are benign, mushroomlike growths in the
colon. People who have one polyp will probably develop
more. Polyps are not cancerous themselves, but they
sometimes develop into cancer. Thus, if a doctor discov-
ers a polyp he'll want to check it periodically and, in
some cases, remove it. Polyps often cause no symptoms
at all, but sometimes they bleed, resulting in rectal bleeding or blood in the stool; they may also cause diarrhea or
a discharge of mucus into the stool.

Colon Cancer and Polyps vs. IBS

How can you tell if your symptoms are those of IBS and
not colon cancer or polyps? Sometimes you can't, which
is why it's essential to get a doctor's diagnosis. But
sometimes there are distinguishing features:

—IBS rarely, if ever, involves blood in the stool or from
the rectum.

—Fatigue, weight loss, and diminished appetite may be associated with colon cancer but not with IBS.

—Rectal pain, associated with colon cancer, is rarely seen with IBS.

A Word of Warning

None of this information is intended to frighten you. Even if some of your symptoms match those described above, don't assume you have cancer or some other serious disease. It's precisely because these conditions mimic each other so closely that you need an expert's opinion. Use the material in this chapter to review your own situation, so you can answer your doctor's questions accurately, and perhaps ask him a few questions of your own.

CONCLUSION

Some of the examinations and tests described in this chapter may sound rather unpleasant, if not downright embarrassing, but they're essential to an accurate diagnosis. Once you and your doctor know for certain your symptoms are those of IBS, you can get down to the business of treatment, and learning how you can take charge of your life.

PART II
TREATING IBS

Your IBS treatment should have three basic goals:

—Symptom relief
—Identification and change of triggering factors
—Finding ways of living with IBS

One of the most important factors in the successful treatment of IBS is the relationship you have with your physician. Your doctor should be serious and sympathetic; you should feel comfortable asking him or her any questions you may have. Remember, however, that one of the goals of therapy is to help you adapt to your condition, and to live a normal life independent of the doctor. Try to keep your questions and comments brief and to the point, and don't be put off if the physician recommends certain therapies that you can perform yourself. Remember, the idea is to help you regain control of your life.

On the other hand, don't try anything without your doctor's approval first. If you learn of a new diet, a drug, a support group, or any other means of treatment, ask your doctor before you try it. This is not to receive "permission," but to make sure you're not doing anything harmful. In short, your doctor is not your parent, your conscience, or your captive audience. He is your partner in therapy.

FOUR

FOOD: FRIEND
OR FOE?

"One man's meat is another man's poison." How true this is for the person with IBS! Your best friend lives on coffee; even the smell of it makes you sick. Your husband starts each day with bacon and eggs; you've yet to find a breakfast that won't land you in the bathroom within a few minutes. Or perhaps your sister, who also has IBS, eats chocolate every day, while you can only watch with envy.

All this illustrates one of the most exasperating features of IBS: reactions to food vary among different people, and even within the same person at different times. This is why experts may offer guidelines for choosing appropriate foods, but they can't provide some list of "safe" or "forbidden" foods that applies to everybody.

If you believe that you've somehow caused your IBS by eating certain foods, take heart: food does not cause IBS. That it may aggravate your symptoms is, however, beyond doubt: according to one survey, physicians reported that twenty-five percent of their patients complained that food intensified their stomach pains. Some patients claimed that the very act of eating, particularly breakfast, brought on diarrhea almost immediately.

Why Does Eating Make
IBS Worse?

This may happen for several reasons:

—*Emotions.* Perhaps a certain food or foods have an emotional connotation for you. Maybe the food was served frequently in your household when you were growing up. If mealtimes were times of arguments or anxiety, perhaps you learned to associate certain foods with stress. Or perhaps you saw someone close to you eat the same or a similar food and get sick from it.

—*Exaggerated reflex.* Even in people without IBS, the very act of eating triggers reflex contractions in the colon. No one knows why this happens, but some experts speculate that it may involve the amount of fat in the meal. Normally the gastrocolic reflex, as it is called, begins soon after you start eating, and many people feel the urge to defecate within thirty to sixty minutes after the meal. The contractions start to subside about fifty minutes after you've eaten.

But if you have IBS, your gut is overly sensitive to whatever stimuli are present. You may experience a much more intense gastrocolic reflex that lasts longer and grows stronger, instead of diminishing after an hour or so. Thus you'll feel pain and may have diarrhea, not because of the food you've eaten, but because you've eaten at all.

—*Food allergies and intolerance.* True food allergies, defined by doctors as an overreaction of the immune system to certain components in food, are actually rare among people with IBS. It's possible that food intolerance, or the inability to digest some kinds of food, is present, but so far doctors don't have enough evidence to determine this for sure. The one exception, lactose intolerance, is discussed below.

What's more likely is that IBS patients may have food sensitivities,* in which the digestive system overreacts to some component in certain kinds of food, with cramps, gas, nausea, and indigestion as the result. Caffeine, for example, stimulates intestinal contractions, so after a cup of coffee an IBS sufferer may feel as though her gut is being tied up in knots. Fatty foods initiate the release of the hormone CCK, which also causes GI contractions. Some kinds of fiber increase the production of intestinal gas, leading to pain that may have you doubled over. Even the artificial sweetener sorbitol has been linked to flare-ups in some people, thanks to colon bacteria that metabolize this compound and produce excess gas, leading to pain, bloating, and diarrhea. These symptoms disappear when sorbitol disappears from the diet.

In general, IBS patients report sensitivity to one or more of the following:

—milk and dairy products

—colas

—chocolate

—corn or corn cereals

—eggs

—soybeans

—nuts: peanuts, walnuts, pecans

—citrus fruits or juices

---

*Some experts use the terms *food intolerance* and *food sensitivity* interchangeably to say that certain foods disagree with certain people, regardless of the reason.

—tomatoes

—wheat products

—cinnamon

—pork

—beets

—onion

—garlic

—white potatoes

—fish

—coffee or tea

—shrimp

—bananas

In a study conducted in 1985, British physicians asked 122 IBS patients which foods most frequently triggered their symptoms. Only five percent were sensitive to one food alone, while thirty-two percent reported sensitivities to eleven or more foods.

—*Lactose intolerance.* Lactose intolerance is the inability to digest lactose, the sugar found in milk and many dairy products. Like IBS, the symptoms of lactose intolerance include cramps, gas, diarrhea, and stomach bloating.

Almost one third of the people who report symptoms of IBS are found to have lactose intolerance instead. Among people with IBS as many as forty percent may be lactose intolerant as well. So if your symptoms flare after you consume dairy foods, this may be the cause, or at least a contributor to your woes.

People may differ in their degree of lactose intolerance; some react only after sizable quantities of lactose-containing foods, like one or more glasses of milk, while others can't even put milk in their coffee without experiencing symptoms. In addition, milk products vary in the amount of lactose they contain. Cheese and yogurt have less lactose than milk and may be safely tolerated by some people who cannot drink milk.

Remember, although many people with IBS have lactose intolerance, it is not true of everyone with IBS, and not all lactose-intolerant people have IBS. How can you determine which condition you have? In general, people with lactose intolerance develop symptoms whenever they ingest lactose, while people with IBS react to those foods only when certain other conditions are present, like when they're tired or under stress. If you suspect that you are lactose intolerant, for two weeks try avoiding the dairy products that give you problems and see if your symptoms subside. To confirm the diagnosis your doctor may administer a lactose-intolerance test by having you drink milk on an empty stomach. He may also have you continue the lactose-free diet under his supervision.

If your doctor says you have lactose intolerance, you can easily end your symptoms by avoiding milk and most other dairy products. A registered dietician can tell you how to compensate for the lack of dairy products with other foods. For more information ask your doctor or call the American Dietetic Association, whose address and phone number are given in Chapter Seven.

HOW DIET CAN HELP YOU

Food can be a means of relief as well as an agent of misery. Through wise meal-planning and the right food choices you can eliminate many of the problems you may have come to associate with food. Perhaps the most important dietary changes you can make are to increase your intake of fiber, and decrease your intake of fat. These measures have health benefits beyond helping you avoid IBS flare-ups; they'll also lower your risk of cancer and heart disease. Indeed, a diet lower in fat and higher in fiber has been endorsed by the American Cancer Society and the American Heart Association for precisely those reasons. These are changes everyone can live with.

Fiber Options

Adding fiber to your diet may be the single most helpful factor in treating your IBS, according to some experts.

Fiber is the indigestible part of many plant foods, including fruits, vegetables, and grains. Because it cannot be broken down and absorbed in the small intestine, fiber passes right into the large intestine and out with the stool.

But even though it's not digested, fiber plays an important role in maintaining health. It attaches to chemicals in food and the digestive tract and helps carry them out of the body; in some cases these chemicals are thought to cause cancer if allowed to remain in the GI tract. Fiber also makes the intestinal muscles work to push it through, thus exercising those muscles and keeping them in good working tone. Finally, fiber absorbs water and hastens the transit time of waste through the colon, preventing the formation of the hard, dry stool usually associated with constipation. Fiber also helps prevent diarrhea by absorbing much of the excess water that is part of a loose bowel movement. And it promotes regularity by helping the GI muscles work properly and by keeping the GI tract mildly distended, which prevents spasms.

Currently Americans consume fifteen to twenty grams of fiber each day (there are twenty-eight grams of fiber in one ounce). The National Cancer Institute recommends we raise that intake to twenty-five to thirty-five grams each day. This is often difficult to do, however, particularly for people with IBS, so doctors usually tell their IBS patients to eat just enough fiber to produce soft stools that are easily passed. Easy does it is the best rule of thumb to follow when trying to eat more fiber; if you add too much too soon, gas and other symptoms may actually get worse. The gradual addition of bran or other high-fiber foods over a period of several weeks is the best way to proceed.

The foods highest in fiber include:

—broccoli, cabbage, Brussels sprouts
—onions
—corn
—carrots
—beets
—celery
—cauliflower
—potatoes with skin
—dried fruits: prunes, raisins, apricots
—fresh apricots
—oranges
—strawberries and blackberries
—lentils and kidney beans
—whole grains, including oats, brown rice, and whole wheat

Some tips to remember when trying to add more fiber to your diet:

1. Whenever possible, consume fruits in their whole form rather than as juice. A whole apple, for example, contains far more fiber than a glass of apple juice.

2. Oat bran has received a lot of publicity recently because of evidence that it reduces cholesterol along with all its other health benefits. You can add oat bran to your diet by sprinkling it on yogurt, cottage cheese, or fruit salad, or by eating muffins or breads baked with oat bran. And, of course, there's always oat cereal like oatmeal. Some doctors recommend a therapeutic dose of ten to twenty-five grams of oat bran each day (a bowl of oatmeal contains about twenty-eight grams), but your gut is your ultimate guide: if that dose elicits persistent symptoms, take what's most convenient and comfortable for you.

3. Give yourself four to six weeks to adjust to your new fiber-full diet. If your gas and feelings of distension do not diminish in this period of time, your doctor may have you try a natural fiber laxative, which may produce less gas. Sometimes you can start with a laxative product and then, once you're used to that, graduate to bran and other high-fiber foods. A small percentage of IBS patients, however, simply cannot tolerate more than minimal amounts of dietary fiber.

4. When increasing fiber intake, be sure to drink plenty of water: six to eight eight-ounce glasses each day.

Fat Facts

Often you can minimize or even eliminate your symptoms by eating less fat. More than any other nutrient, fat stimulates strong colon contractions, possibly because it leads to the release of CCK, or possibly for other reasons. Fatty foods also contain more calories than any other kind of food, so if you get cramps or the runs after a heavy, greasy meal, this could have as much to do with the number of calories you've consumed as the amount of fat. High-fat foods include:

—butter, margarine, and oils such as olive or peanut oil

—shortening

—bacon or sausage

—nondairy whipped toppings

—whole milk, cream, ice cream

—chocolate

—poultry skin

—foods fried in a lot of butter or grease; anything deep-fried

—nuts and nut butters, like peanut butter

—cream cheese and many hard cheeses

—certain cuts of red meat

"Stop!" you may be thinking. "You're naming all my favorite foods!" Unfortunately, you may be right. Nutritionists know that a food's fat content has a lot to do with its palatability. What's more, most high-fat foods are also high in sugar or salt, two other ingredients known to improve taste. If you were to ask people to name their favorite food, chances are it would be something high in fat.

But you don't have to be a slave to your taste buds. Many IBS patients have learned to satisfy their hunger and their desire for something special or "forbidden" with starchy foods such as pasta, rice, and bread. If it's okay with your colon, these foods make excellent substitutions for items like fried chicken or peanut-butter sandwiches. Small quantities of high-fat condiments like butter or creamy sauces are all right as long as they don't elicit flare-ups. Or you can experiment with some low-fat sauces like tomato or marinara.

If you like milk and aren't lactose intolerant, try skim milk and skim milk products, like ice milk and low-fat cottage cheese. Instead of fried chicken, substitute broiled or roasted chicken without the skin—ditto for turkey. If you have a sweet tooth, train yourself to reach for the fruit bowl instead of a box of chocolates.

Along with relieving your symptoms, lowering your intake of fat may have a bonus: you'll lose weight! Ounce for ounce, fat has more than twice the calories of protein or carbohydrate. If you make some of the changes suggested here, you may easily find yourself dropping pounds.

In addition to eating more fiber and less fat, you can change your diet in other ways that may increase your relief. The lists below includes the most popular and effective tips. Remember, however, that these are just suggestions. What works for you may not work for anyone else, and what works for your best friend may not work for you. Be patient; experiment by adding or eliminating foods until you discover what's best for you. And it's a good idea to consult your doctor or a qualified nutritionist or dietician if you plan to make any drastic changes in your diet.

FOOD TIPS TO MANAGE IBS

1. Always account for your total caloric needs when you plan your daily food intake.

2. Select the most nutritious foods possible. Avoid highly processed convenience foods, which are often high in fat.

3. Eliminate the foods that disagree with you and, whenever possible, choose acceptable foods from the same food group. For example, among vegetables, cabbage may be a disaster, while spinach is perfectly fine.

4. Don't exclude any food that you like and can tolerate.

5. Change the texture or consistency of foods to discover what you can and can't tolerate. A whole orange may be forbidden, but orange juice may be all right.

6. To ensure variety prepare your food through any acceptable method.

7. Chew your food slowly and thoroughly.

8. If necessary, when you eat out or with friends and family, have on hand a list of foods you must avoid.

9. Make sure your food is at moderate temperature. Very cold foods in particular may elicit intestinal spasms and pain.

10. Pureeing raw fruits and vegetables makes them easier to digest.

11. Make sure your daily diet includes at least one serving of a citrus fruit or fruit juice, a dark green vegetable, and a dark yellow or orange fruit or vegetable (example: carrots, yellow squash).

12. Exercise helps you relax and digest your food better.

13. If your diet is highly restricted, consult a registered dietician to see how you can best meet your nutritional needs.

The next two recommendations are so important that they deserve a detailed explanation.

14. *Eat small, frequent meals instead of two or three big meals.* Many IBS patients say they feel better when they eat four to six small snacks instead of fewer, larger meals, even if the total number of calories is the same. This may have something to do with gut hormones, which are released in response to food and cause intestinal contractions. A smaller quantity of food perhaps elicits a smaller quantity of hormone, with milder effects on the gut.

15. *Make mealtimes pleasant.* Remember Sheila, who discussed her symptoms in Chapter One? Her doctor asked her to describe mealtimes in her house when she was growing up. "We had a very close family," she recalled. "My parents, my sister, my brother, and I had dinner together every night—that was the rule." Her doctor prodded a little more, however, and Sheila's memory improved. "My father would use that time to discuss major family issues, and to talk about what we'd learned at school. He'd go around the table and ask each one of us kids some ridiculous math question, or something that had been in the news that day, or about a book we were reading in school. If any of us gave the wrong answer, he would sit there and grill us and usually end

up giving us a lecture on how we had to study harder. Then he'd turn to my mother and start asking her about the bills or telling her about some problem he was having at work." By this time she was in tears. "You know," she said, "my father came home every day around six, and by five-thirty my stomach would be riding a roller coaster. We had this myth of a close, harmonious family, but the fact is I hated it every night we had to eat together."

It seems too simple to be true, but a leisurely, genuinely harmonious atmosphere while you eat may be one of your most powerful weapons against IBS. In a recent study conducted in Philadelphia, by Dr. Donald R. Morse of the Temple University School of Dentistry, twelve dental hygiene students were subjected to "stress" conditions and "relaxed" conditions before eating a breakfast of Cheerios. In the "stress" condition the students had to solve a math problem in their heads, starting five minutes before the meal and continuing as they ate. In the "relaxed" condition the students meditated before and during breakfast. As a measure of the stress they were experiencing, their heart rates and blood pressure levels were monitored, as was another parameter of stress known as the galvanic skin response. The result: Digestion was more rapid when the subjects were relaxed. According to Dr. Morse these findings demonstrated that life-style and intestinal disorders may be linked.

Our society abounds with obstacles to relaxed eating. Even when we take the time to eat we often eat while reading or watching TV. A busy restaurant may hustle you out as soon as you've had your last swallow to make room for the people waiting at the bar.

Or, as in Sheila's family, some people mistake a "close, harmonious" family dinnertime with an opportunity to discuss all the unpleasant things that happened during the day.

More often than not, however, the problem boils down to one of time. So many of us are always in a rush: we bolt breakfast, lunch at our desks, grab dinner on the run. How many people do you know who never eat breakfast at all? Some individuals thrive on such a pace, but the person with IBS deserves a kinder, gentler routine. Do yourself a favor: review your daily activities and think of ways you can create a more favorable climate in which to eat. This may involve getting up a few minutes earlier to have breakfast, or perhaps preparing breakfast or some part of it the night before. Whenever possible, take a full hour for lunch and eat outside your office—even if it's just a brown-bag lunch in an empty conference room. If there's time left, take a stroll, do some window-shopping. Take the same care with dinner: even if you live alone, you can work in some time to prepare something you enjoy and eat it in surroundings that make you feel pampered and relaxed. Invest in a microwave oven if you don't like spending a long time over the stove. And if you're really too rushed to shop or cook, stop off for some take-out, or have food delivered in.

This is one of the many subjective aspects of IBS. If too many of your meals are gobbled on the run, ask yourself what you need to slow down, relax, and feel good. Then try to provide that for yourself. The difference it makes in your symptoms could be astounding.

THE ADDS DIET FOR PEOPLE WITH DIGESTIVE DISORDERS

Thus far most of the suggestions in this chapter have been fairly general in nature. If you're looking for more specific tips on how to discover exactly which foods to avoid, the American Digestive Disease Society (ADDS) has published *ADDS Dietary Plans,* a booklet explaining in detail how you can learn which foods are your enemies. It also offers several dietary plans for people who are sensitive to certain categories of food. Most of the information in this section comes from that book, which you can obtain from ADDS at the address given in Chapter Seven.

Be a Diet Detective

The best way to take charge of your condition and your life is to play an active role in discovering and changing the factors that complicate your health. Think of food as a suspect in the crime of making you sick, and gather as many clues as you can to find the culprit(s). As for the culinary innocent bystanders, ADDS recommends that you develop a "food pool," defined as nutritious foods you enjoy and can eat with impunity. You can devise a food pool fairly easily by keeping a food diary for two weeks, from which you determine what items are safe for you and can be part of your food pool. The most effective diaries include this information:

—what you ate or drank
—when you had it

—how it was prepared and the temperature at which it was consumed
—how much you had
—the emotional climate in which you consumed it
—any symptoms you associate with that food or beverage, including their severity and duration

A detailed record of your symptoms can also help you pinpoint exactly which foods are no-nos for you. The details you might consider recording include:

—pain: when, where in your body, and the nature of the pain (sudden and severe? dull and "achy?" intermittent or steady?)
—stool: the idea of inspecting your stool may seem embarrassing or even disgusting, but doctors can determine a lot from the appearance of a bowel movement, and so can you. A pale, putty-colored stool suggests problems digesting fat, while black stool may mean the presence of blood or too many iron supplements. If you see mucus, which looks like raw egg white, it may mean the colon is irritated from an infection or an allergy, while a frothy stool forcefully expelled and smelling of vinegar suggests a problem digesting starch. If you can associate an unusual bowel movement with other symptoms and a particular food, you may be able to attain at least partial relief.
—weight: a weekly weight record helps you keep track of upward or downward trends that you might otherwise not detect. Loss of weight may suggest the presence of Crohn's disease or ulcerative colitis, while weight gain suggests you're eating too many calories or not exercising enough—or maybe a little of both.

—medicine: some medicines may influence your symptoms, so if you want a truly accurate picture you may wish to discuss with your doctor the possibility of temporarily discontinuing some or all of the medicines you may be taking.

Tracking the Guilty Party

The Sam Spades of the IBS world may wish to pursue their investigations further by conducting a food test. If you've narrowed your list of suspects to just a few foods, you may be able to extract a confession through following these steps:

1. Eliminate just one of the suspicious foods from your diet for at least four days. If you test more than one food at a time, you won't know which one is causing your symptoms.

2. After that, eat that food *only* for one or two days—not more! Have a normal portion at first. If no symptoms occur, have half a portion one hour later. If there's still no reaction, have another normal portion of the food at your next regular mealtime. If, on this regimen, you haven't experienced symptoms within six hours, chances are the food is probably safe for you.

3. Try the food in its purest form. Eggs, for example, should be eaten poached or soft boiled, rather than scrambled or fried because this requires the addition of butter and sometimes milk. If wheat is your suspect, have it in the form of a cereal—like cream of wheat (not too hot), or puffed or shredded wheat—but omit milk, sugar, and butter.

4. Get your doctor's permission to conduct this test. Under no circumstances should you maintain this diet for more than two days, because it is extremely unbalanced.

5. If, after two days, you haven't had a bad reaction to the food, you can assume it's okay to include in your food pool. If, on the other hand, you react violently within an hour the first time you try it, there's no reason to continue the test—the food is one to avoid.

6. If you want to test more than one food, wait at least a few weeks between tests.

IN CONCLUSION

Thousands of pages have been written on the subject of diet and IBS, but their basic messages are these: Be patient; plan relaxed, leisurely meals; learn what you can and cannot eat; and try adding more fiber.

We'll close this chapter with two notes of caution:

1. Don't go overboard when eliminating food from your diet. If more than a few foods trigger your symptoms, see a doctor and a dietician for their advice. Otherwise, you risk having a diet so limited or unbalanced that you may develop nutritional deficiencies.

2. Remember that food is not the only culprit when it comes to IBS. If your symptoms don't respond to dietary changes alone, don't despair. There are other things you can try, like stress-coping techniques or medication.

DRUG THERAPY FOR IBS: WHAT HELPS, WHAT DOESN'T

Drug treatment of IBS is controversial. Some doctors believe that patients respond more to the physician's attention and reassurance than to any particular medication. This has been borne out by studies in which one group of IBS patients were given an actual drug, while another received a placebo. More than half the IBS patients in these studies responded to the placebo—in some instances the figure was as high as eighty percent; that is, their symptoms abated. In fact, few medicines have been shown to be superior to a placebo in the treatment of IBS. Thus, many experts believe that some patients respond as much to the power of suggestion as they do to any drug.

Are Drugs Ever Appropriate?

Nevertheless, many doctors do prescribe drugs of one kind or another for their patients with IBS. There are some situations in which medicine may be called for:

—For the treatment of specific symptoms, such as pain or diarrhea.

—If the patient doesn't respond to any other form of therapy.

—If the patient is severely agitated or depressed.

—In some cases, to allow the patient some initial relief for her symptoms, and to give her time to learn how to manage her condition herself.

What Your Doctor Should Know

If your doctor does prescribe medication for you, make sure he knows if you:

—have recently had a heart attack

—have glaucoma

—have a history of diabetes, epilepsy, or other form of seizure disorder

—have heart disease, an enlarged prostate gland, or an overactive thyroid gland

—regularly take any other drugs, even if you don't need a prescription to buy them

—are pregnant, nursing a baby, or trying to become pregnant

—have any drug allergies

—plan to have any surgery that requires general anesthesia

—smoke cigarettes

—drink alcohol heavily or regularly

—like to sit in the sun (some drugs make your skin overly sensitive to sunlight) or in a sauna (other products may affect your ability to sweat and adapt to extreme heat; this could lead to heat stroke)

—have any other digestive disorders, such as ulcerative colitis
—cannot empty your bladder completely
—have bronchitis, asthma, emphysema, a hiatal hernia, myasthenia gravis, liver disease, or kidney disease
—are on a special diet

What to Ask Your Doctor

Before taking any drug make sure you ask some important questions:

—Is this drug available in generic form? Generic drugs are less expensive than their brand-name equivalents.
—Is the prescription refillable?
—When is the best time for me to take this drug? If I must take it more than two or three times a day, do I have to get up in the middle of the night to take it?
—What are the side effects of this drug? (A side effect is an unanticipated reaction to the product that may or may not be harmful.)

MEDICINES USED MOST FREQUENTLY IN THE TREATMENT OF IBS

Doctors who use drugs to help treat IBS usually prescribe one or more of these:

Bulk Laxatives

The active ingredient in a bulk laxative is fiber, which fights constipation naturally by exercising the digestive tract and helping the stool retain water. Bulk laxatives are available without a prescription; one example is Metamucil.

No other laxative is recommended for the treatment of IBS. In fact, many people overuse laxatives and become dependent on them, upsetting GI function and, ironically, often triggering the symptoms of IBS. Abuse of nonbulk laxatives sometimes leads to tolerance and persistent constipation that can be alleviated only with higher doses of the laxative. In high enough doses laxatives may have such side effects as skin rashes, severe cramps, and general derangement of one's body chemistry. Nerve damage in the colon may result from the prolonged, heavy use of laxatives, leaving a bloated, constipated organ that responds only to artificial stimuli. This condition is diminished when the patient weans himself off the laxative.

Antidiarrheals, Anticholinergics,*
or Antispasmodics

These products relieve digestive-tract symptoms through their action on the nerves of the GI tract. Despite their different names their functions basically overlap. The names are, however, self-descriptive, for the primary function of these drugs is to relieve intestinal spasms

*An anticholinergic is a drug that inhibits the action of nerves called cholinergic nerves, because they secrete a substance known as acetylcholine.

and their attendant cramps and diarrhea. Some doctors question the efficacy of these drugs for most of these purposes, saying their only real use is for the relief of pain.

Some of the drug names you may hear are: Antrenyl, Banthine, Pathilon, Quarzan, Donnagel, Lomotil, or Barbadonna.

Most of the side effects associated with these products reflect their action on the nervous system: blurred vision, dry mouth and throat, constipation, impaired urination, hives or a skin rash, dizziness, confusion, and delirium. The skin and mental symptoms are, however, rare.

Tranquilizers

If a doctor believes a patient is seriously anxious or agitated, he may prescribe a tranquilizer, of which Valium is probably the best known. Tranquilizers provide temporary relief of anxiety and may help break the cycle of stress-anxiety-symptoms-more-stress that some IBS patients experience.

Not all doctors recommend tranquilizers for IBS, however. Many fear their patients may use these drugs as a substitute for developing coping skills, and there is the very real danger of addiction. At best, tranquilizers may calm you temporarily, allow you to gain a more balanced perspective on your condition, and give you time to get your symptoms under control through other means, like changes in diet. Under no circumstances should they be used on a regular basis in the treatment of IBS.

Antidepressants

Most experts agree that IBS is not necessarily a psychosomatic disorder, because many—some would say most—patients with IBS have perfectly healthy personalities. There is, however, one emotional or psychological condition that has been definitely linked with IBS: depression. When the depression is treated, the symptoms of IBS diminish.

It's normal to be sad or depressed after the death of a loved one, a divorce, the loss of a job, or other traumatic events. Eventually, however, these feelings decrease and the individual gets on with life. But with clinical depression the feelings persist indefinitely and the sadness is far more intense. Some people get depressed from having to live with a chronic disease like lupus, rheumatoid arthritis, or even IBS—in these cases a circular pattern may occur in which the depression occurs in response to the disease, the patient is less likely to care for herself so she feels worse, which intensifies the depression, etcetera, etcetera. But sometimes there is no triggering event; hopeless feelings just settle in like a fog on a rainy night—only, this fog doesn't lift.

The symptoms of clinical depression include:

—a history of clinical depression in your family
—a depressed, irritable, or anxious mood that persists despite any attempts at cheering up
—unexplainable aches and pains
—the fear that you are going crazy or that disaster lies just around the corner
—feeling emotionally numb; the inability to experience normal emotions like joy, grief, or pleasure; the feeling that the world is empty or drab

—a loss of interest in activities you used to enjoy

—the inability to concentrate

—unfounded feelings of guilt or indecisiveness

—withdrawal from social activities

—feeling that life is hopeless or that you are helpless to change things; a generally pessimistic outlook

—insomnia

—persistent, recurrent thoughts of suicide or death

—sleep problems: difficulty falling asleep, waking up frequently during the night, or awakening too early in the morning and not being able to go back to sleep

—loss of appetite and weight

—loss of sexual desire

—if you are woman, menstrual irregularities

—the tendency to put yourself down

This list may seem pretty depressing in itself, but fortunately depression can be treated. When depression is compounded by IBS, some doctors prescribe antidepressants along with other forms of medication, but some antidepressants may relieve GI symptoms as well.

Among the more popular antidepressants are Elavil, Tofranil, Pamelor, Adapin, and Sinequan. These products can do enormous good, but they must be used with care. Constipation is one of their potential side effects, which may only make things worse for someone with IBS. Other possible side effects include drowsiness or light-headedness, dry mouth, and problems with urination. If your doctor prescribes an antidepressant, he may have you return regularly to monitor the drug's level in your blood and any individual reactions you may experience. An optimal dose for one person may be dangerously high or ineffectively low for someone else.

Prokinetics

The newest drugs on the IBS horizon are prokinetic drugs, which are thought to affect GI motility. While some doctors have prescribed these compounds already, knowledge about them is still in its infancy, and many physicians feel that more research should be done.

DRUG THERAPY: IS IT FOR YOU?

In all likelihood the most powerful remedy your doctor will prescribe will be some bran or a bulk laxative. Drugs may be used to treat a specific symptom, such as pain, or an underlying condition, like depression, but most doctors today agree that drugs play only a minor role, if any, in the long-term management of IBS.

IBS responds best to the control you exert by learning what situations trigger your symptoms and how you can change things for the better. Many physicians are reluctant to prescribe too many drugs for fear that this may prevent patients from helping themselves. On the other hand, when the pain is severe or the diarrhea just won't stop, it's nice to know that relief is available.

LESS STRESS!

What is stress?

Ask ten different people, you'll get ten different answers. It's a busy day at work or an uncooperative spouse. It's rushing to meet a plane, a deadline, a friend; it's tolerating a week at your mother-in-law's. It could be as minor as a boring movie or as major as the death of a loved one or a cross-country move.

Nor does stress have to be negative. Getting married, finding a better job, or moving to a bigger house are also forms of stress. You may not perceive them as such, but they may require just as much wear and tear on the body as do less pleasant situations.

The best answer, then, to the question "What is stress?" is that stress is an unavoidable part of life. Stress research began in earnest roughly fifty years ago, and many writers on the subject claim that "modern life" is inordinately stressful. It is impossible to know for sure if cavemen fighting saber-toothed tigers or medieval vassals toiling at the whim of their overlords experienced less stress than we do today, but it is certainly true that stress affects all of us, and eventually extracts a price.

There are two basic forms of stress. One involves a major change in your life, such as moving, getting married, or the death of a spouse. The second form is more subtle. It has to do with the daily circumstances that conspire to keep you just a little off balance: never knowing when a difficult boss will snap, hoping a child's grades will improve, making sure a dinner party is a success, etcetera. The end result of this kind of stress is similar in nature, if not degree, to the conditions imposed by a bigger change, because it demands adaptation to unfamiliar or uncertain circumstances. It also reminds you that despite your best efforts, certain things are simply beyond your control. So it's not surprising that the most popular stress-reduction techniques emphasize relaxation and gaining more control over your life.

Stress Takes a Toll

Stress may be part of a full and active life, but persistent, unrelieved stress may push body systems to the point where one or more of them break down. For this reason it has been suggested that stress should sometimes be considered a chronic disease. Again, remember that stressful events may be happy ones as well as sad. If you get engaged, win a promotion, hear from a long-lost brother, buy a new car, learn your brother is going to Harvard, and redecorate your home all within the space of six months, don't be surprised if your symptoms flare up. One rule of thumb you might use when considering the degree of stress involved with a certain event is to assess how much this event will change your daily routine, and thus how much adaptive or coping behavior you'll need to handle it.

What Constitutes a Major Stress?

If you turn back to the questionnaire that ended Chapter One, you'll find that Question #7 included a long list of events and asked how many you had experienced over the last two years. That list was developed in 1967 by Thomas H. Holmes and Richard H. Rahe, a psychiatrist and psychologist at the University of Washington in Seattle. The Holmes-Rahe scale, as it is now known, lists the social events requiring change and adjustment in life patterns that were most frequently associated with illness. To refresh your memory, the ten most stress events were (in descending order):

—the death of a spouse
—divorce
—marital separation
—jail term
—death of close family member
—personal injury or illness
—marriage
—being fired at work
—marital reconciliation
—retirement

This list is now widely used to determine the amount of stress someone has experienced recently. It is not, however, exhaustive. Other major forms of negative stress include:

—pain
—illness

—surgery

—a wound or a burn

—an infection

—living in a very hot or humid climate

—exposure to pollution, radiation, or toxic compounds

Fight or Flight?

Stress affects you physically, so while you can tolerate temporary instances of intense stress, recurrent episodes of stress will wear you down.

When the brain perceives a stressful situation, it tells a gland called the adrenal medulla to release hormones called catecholamines, one of which is adrenaline (most American scientists refer to it as epinephrine). Adrenaline affects almost every organ in the body, including the eyes, lungs, heart, muscles, and vital organs, preparing you to flee a dangerous situation or to stand your ground and fight. Your pulse quickens, you breathe faster, your blood sugar rises, and the circulation to your legs increases in case you have to run. Physiologists refer to this condition as the "fight or flight" reaction.

Unfortunately our physical evolution has been much slower than our social development. The fight-or-flight response is best suited to a world in which hungry lions or tigers lurked around the next bend, waiting for their unsuspecting prey, or in which a warrior from a neighboring tribe might take a stab at heroism by taking a stab at you.

The dangers of today's world usually take a different form. Waiting in slow-moving traffic when you're already late for work, hoping you can pay all your bills on time, praying that your son's Mohawk hairdo grows out before your mother comes to visit—these are all forms of stress, to be sure, but they don't require the physical changes you need when you have to fight or flee. Still, our bodies have as yet developed no other response to stress, so the physical effects of being gridlocked while the clock ticks away are similar to, but less intense than, those of being threatened by an enemy. But there's an important difference: once you escape the lion, you can relax and recover your equilibrium. But rush-hour traffic, a slim wallet, or a difficult child are things you must endure every day. Without appropriate mechanisms for relaxing or coping with stress, the wear and tear of daily life slowly erodes your health and well-being.

Signs of Stress

The signs that you may be overly stressed or may have difficulty handling stress include:

—nervous twitches or tics, such as twitchy eyelids

—frequent headaches or colds

—dry mouth

—poor posture

—pain in the chest, shoulder, joints, or lower back

—irritability while waiting in line or in a crowd

—self-destructive habits, such as smoking, excessive drinking, overeating, or insufficient physical exercise

—dramatic changes in behavior—obsessive neatness in a normally messy person, for example

—sudden outbursts of emotion, such as anger or joy

—difficulty expressing anger

—indecisiveness

—pessimism, worrying a lot

—feeling that you're helpless, that your life is out of control

IBS and Stress

Stress does not cause IBS, and many people cannot relate their symptoms to any stressful events at all. Many others, however, know that the first sign of stress will turn their guts to ice. Among the events IBS patients most frequently associate with their symptoms are:

—marital discord

—worries about family

—financial difficulty

—problems on the job

—fatigue combined with stress, the wrong kind of food, or some other troublesome factor

—a combination of relatively minor stresses, such as a deadline plus a business trip, or anxiety plus too many cups of coffee

How are changes in emotional state translated into intestinal symptoms? As yet, no one knows for sure. That this happens at all is not surprising, because chemicals made in the intestine, such as CCK, are also made in the brain, and situations involving anxiety or fear do evoke changes in digestive-tract function, even in people who don't have IBS. In one study seventy percent of the participants without IBS reported bowel symptoms in response to stressful situations. In people with IBS the symptoms are more frequent and more intense.

The anxiety and depression that frequently accompany extreme stress may lead to symptoms in any body system, and some experts note that stress may contribute to such serious conditions as lupus, diabetes, myasthenia gravis, or even leukemia. If some people respond to stress with symptoms of IBS, it may simply be that the gut is their most vulnerable spot. People with different vulnerabilities may develop migraine headaches or asthma.

Discussing the relationship between stress and IBS requires some delicacy. If it's presented in the wrong light you may think, "So it *is* all in my head. I'm just a neurotic hypochondriac," when this isn't the case at all. In fact, some studies indicate that people with IBS are less likely than others to report certain forms of pain. All of us have different ways of coping with stress, and in the IBS patient the digestive tract seems to be the vehicle for reflecting or discharging the tension in life. But to tell someone with IBS that her symptoms are all her own fault or all in her head is like telling the asthmatic that she's not really suffocating, or the migraine sufferer that she can will her pain away.

COPING WITH STRESS

IBS patients do have certain characteristics suggesting that their digestive symptoms are their way of coping with stress. More than other people IBS sufferers report frequent or serious stressful events early in life. There's also evidence that some people have subconsciously learned to use their bowel symptoms as an excuse to take a break when they're tired or under stress, instead of acknowledging the very real need for a vacation. Perhaps you recall Margie, who was quoted in Chapter One as saying that her parents gave her toys and special attention when she was sick. Doctors speculate that, like Margie, many people who received such unwitting reinforcement for their symptoms learned to respond in this way whenever they are under stress.

Clearly, if your episodes of IBS occur in response to stress, one of the best ways to regain control of your life is to learn some stress-coping techniques. Indeed, *what* you do may be less important than the fact that you *do* it, since evidence is mounting that body systems return to normal when patients take an active part in their own care—be it through assertiveness training, meditation, relaxation techniques, or other healthy means of coping.

The First Step

The first step toward taking charge of your body and your life is to commit yourself to changing the aspects of your life that exacerbate stress, and to change your way of dealing with the stress that you can't avoid.

Start by keeping a journal in which you record your symptoms, their duration, when and where they occurred, when they stopped, and the events just prior to their occurrence. You might also add any other relevant information: your emotional state at the time, any illnesses you might have had, any ongoing stresses in your life, and what you ate or drank. After a month or so you'll be able to see patterns in your symptoms and what elicited them; you may also detect certain behavioral patterns that you can change without too much trouble. For example, you may find that mornings are particularly stressful: You always seem to get caught in traffic and arrive late for work. Perhaps you can change this situation by getting up a little earlier, or performing some tasks the night before—putting out your clothes or fixing lunch, to name two. Examine your diary for stressful situations that are relatively easy to change, and use your imagination to help find ways to change them. You may also wish to enlist the aid of family members in this project.

Something else you can learn from a journal is your "cognitive style"—the personal interpretation you place on certain events. Each of us sees the world differently, and occasions you perceive as stressful or annoying may be approached differently by others. For example, here's what one woman wrote:

> August 25: I hate this job! My boss sends me to the post office every day just when the line is longest. If I have to do this one more time I'll go insane! Spent twenty minutes in bathroom after I returned.

Unfortunately, standing in line is an unavoidable part of her job. This lady may not be able to change her job, but she can change her approach by:

—Taking a book with her and reading while waiting in line.

—Performing another work-related task while she's waiting.

—Practicing one of the relaxation techniques described later in this chapter.

—Striking up a conversation with the next person in line. Misery loves company!

—Using the time to make a shopping list or plan her tasks for the next day.

—Buying a personal stereo and listening to music she finds relaxing.

Apply this kind of creative thinking to the other troublesome but unavoidable events in your life, and you may arrive at countless ways of reducing stress.

Here's another example:

> September 20: Woke up seven-thirty. No breakfast. Everything okay until stuck in traffic; half hour late for work. Symptoms began around ten-thirty.

In this instance it's not hard to imagine that this person might save herself a lot of stress if she simply set her alarm to go off a half hour earlier.

Finally, here's an entry from Margie's journal:

> June 25: Just got engaged! Mother and sister thrilled; mother arriving next Saturday to help with plans. To do: start looking for dress, place for reception, silver & china, invitation list, etc., etc., etc. Arrived at work early to complete Johnson report. Lunch with client; ate too much. Got home eight P.M.; symptoms began almost immediately.

In this case Margie should probably try to pace herself. If she knows she's going to be burdened with wedding plans, she should try to lighten her load at work by delegating responsibility to her subordinates. If that's not possible, she should enlist all the wedding help she can from her mother, sister, fiancé, and friends. In any event she should block out plenty of time to rest and practice stress-reduction techniques, since the upcoming months promise to be unusually stressful.

The Negative Internal Monologue

Sometimes changing our responses to stress is as simple as changing our internal monologue—that voice in our head that comments or editorializes on everything. Perhaps now, while waiting on line, your inner voice is saying, "What a drag. I've at least ten people ahead of me. Why can't that woman up front put the stamps on her envelopes before she comes to the post office? Why is the person waiting on her so slow? And of course three of the windows are closed completely—typical. This task is beneath my abilities anyway—Mr. Jones probably makes me do it because he thinks I can't do anything else. Maybe I can't do anything else. My work really isn't what it could be—there was that time I screwed up last week and the mistake I made yesterday. Maybe I really can't do anything better. . . ." See how it works?

Now try changing the script: "How nice to be out of the office for a few minutes! You really see a cross section of humanity at the post office. That poor woman up front has so much mail, she couldn't even figure out how much postage she'd need for it all—now she's even got the clerk confused. I'm glad I get this opportunity to stretch my legs in the middle of the day—it's not healthy to spend the whole day sitting behind a desk. I guess Mr.

Jones must think I've got my work under control if he lets me spend this much time outside the office every day." Corny? Maybe, but you get the idea.

RELAX!

Relaxation is probably the best weapon against the ravages of stress. In addition to familiar ways of relaxing such as taking a warm bath, pursuing a hobby, having a massage, taking a nap, or daydreaming of a soothing scene (psychologists consider napping and daydreaming healthy ways of relieving stress, as long as you don't indulge in them to the point where they disrupt your life), there are many other relaxation techniques you can try. Once you become adept at them you can practice them anywhere, anytime you feel your bowels start to churn.

Tips to Help You Relax

Before you try any of the methods described in this chapter, here are some tips to help get you in the proper mood:

1. Comfort is paramount. Loosen tight clothing and remove any heavy or tight jewelry.

2. Put yourself in surroundings that are quiet and peaceful; you may wish to close the curtains or dim the light.

3. Don't try to force a particular sensation. Instead, merely observe your body's response when you try a particular technique.

4. Allow yourself enough time for the technique to take effect—most experts recommend at least thirty minutes per session.

5. Practice makes perfect. Try these exercises daily at least once a day (many people do them twice a day).

6. Make your mind a blank. If unwanted thoughts occur, let them drift by—don't dwell on them. This may be difficult at first, but the more you practice, the easier it will become. The idea is to remain serene and relaxed.

Relaxation Techniques

This section is meant to acquaint you with relaxation techniques you may not have considered before, and to encourage you to try them or to develop some techniques of your own, based on what you read. If you'd like more information on any of them, some of the books recommended in the bibliography contain excellent discussions of relaxation techniques.

Visualization

Visualization is a lot like daydreaming. As the name implies, you close your eyes and visualize a scene that makes you feel happy and relaxed. Place yourself in the scene: if it's a Swiss mountain village, feel the bracing air, see the winding streets, the houses with window boxes full of colorful flowers; see the mountains, with their green slopes and white peaks; hear the cowbells. If it's a beach scene, feel the warm sun, smell the salt air, hear the waves breaking onshore, and feel the spray as they do. Get into your scene as fully as you can; breathe deeply and exhale slowly as you do so.

Deep Breathing

As suggested in the previous section, you can do this exercise along with another exercise, but it's also helpful on its own.

Many of us have gotten into the habit of shallow breathing, particularly when we're under stress. Deep breathing forces you to slow down and concentrate on your breathing, and refreshes and energizes you by carrying more oxygen to the tissues.

To perform this exercise, simply close your eyes, inhale deeply through your nose, and exhale from the mouth. Do this for three to five minutes, then open your eyes and observe how you feel. To make sure you're breathing deeply enough keep a hand on your abdomen the first few times you practice this. You should feel your stomach and abdomen swell as you inhale; then hold that breath for ten to fifteen seconds, and exhale. Don't do it too quickly, or you'll hyperventilate. Slow and easy does it.

Autogenic Relaxation

This technique is a form of self-hypnosis, in which you repeat a certain instruction to yourself five times and observe your physical reaction. You instruct yourself to feel some relaxing sensation, such as "My hands are heavy and warm," or "My stomach is regular and calm." Ideally you should develop an entire ritual in which you begin by relaxing the muscles in your head and neck and travel down the body to your legs and feet. For maximum benefit this exercise should be done twice a day.

Remember: don't force yourself to feel anything. Your hands may not feel heavy and warm the first time you try this; in fact, it may take a few days of practice before you start to feel the sensations you're after. Praise yourself for taking control of your stress, and keep practicing—you'll get results.

Deep Muscle Relaxation

Developed in the nineteen twenties and thirties, deep muscle relaxation involves tightening each of the body's muscle groups—head, face, hands, arms, legs, etcetera—for about ten seconds, then relaxing them and observing how it feels. As with autogenic relaxation it's best done in sequence, starting at the top and working down. This technique is also called active progressive relaxation.

Passive Progressive Relaxation

In this exercise you relax each muscle group in turn without tensing it first. Many people find that this relieves headaches and lowers their blood pressure, and in some IBS patients it seems to pacify irregular colonic movements.

Biofeedback

Biofeedback involves the use of special equipment to give you immediate feedback on biological processes such as heart rate, muscle tension, and body temperature. The equipment consists of an electronic monitoring device with electrodes. This is generally recommended as the first choice for the IBS patient who wants to learn stress-reduction techniques, but it may prove to be a valuable adjunct to the other exercises discussed. If you'd like more information, contact the Biofeedback Society of America, whose address and phone number are given in Chapter Seven.

BEING ASSERTIVE

Assertiveness has become something of a dirty word. Many people apply it to those angry, pushy individuals who get ahead of you on line, cut you off in traffic, or blow their tops when some demand isn't met. But this isn't being assertive; it's being hostile, aggressive, and just plain nasty.

In fact, being assertive means regaining control of your life in the best possible sense. Assertive people see to it that their needs are met and don't allow other people to manipulate or impose their desires on them. Assertive people also take responsibility for their feelings and accept the consequences of their actions. For example, doing a friend a favor even if it's inconvenient for you isn't being "nice"—it's being passive and unassertive. Passive people may appear nice on the outside, but inwardly they're often seething with anger and resentment at allowing themselves to be manipulated and used. Eventually this rage boils over, often destroying friendships, marriages, or one's health. Clearly, as we have seen, this kind of stress is frequently associated with IBS symptoms.

If passivity is one of your character traits, you may want to think about learning how to give your own needs priority for a change.

How Can I Be More Assertive?

The key to being assertive is to know what your needs are and to communicate them honestly but courteously. If Sally asks you to pick up her kids from school and you can't or don't want to do it, you might say, "I'd love to help you out, but Wednesday at three is really a bad time for me." You can explain if you want to, but it isn't necessary.

On the other hand, being assertive also means knowing when you need help, and asking for it. If you ask Sally to pick up your kids, and she gives you a polite but assertive no, you can ask another friend, arrange to have the children met by a taxi, have the kids wait for you at school or at a friend's house, or, in the worst case, pick them up yourself if there's really no other way. Even when things don't go as planned, you'll know that you tried to take care of yourself, and that alone can be a source of satisfaction.

Many books have been written on the subject of being your own best friend, looking out for yourself, communicating better, and other ways of being assertive. In addition, local schools and community colleges frequently offer courses on this subject. If you repeatedly find your stomach churning while you think, "How did I let so-and-so talk me into this?" or "when she said that, I should have said . . ." a little assertiveness training may be of help.

GETTING ORGANIZED

The other great wellspring of stress is lack of time. Many people feel guilty if they're not constantly busy, so they burden themselves with so many commitments and obligations that they start feeling overwhelmed. This isn't healthy for anybody, but for the person with IBS, time pressure can spell disaster.

How can you regain control of your time? First, by remembering your assertiveness techniques and accurately assessing your needs. If you do your best work when you can walk to your job, build in some time in the morning for that. If you can't go out at night without an afternoon nap, schedule your evenings accordingly. If your doctor's appointment is for Tuesday at five, allow extra time for rush-hour traffic. And if Sally wants you to pick up her kids a half hour later, say no! (Politely, of course.)

Second, get organized. Make shopping lists so you don't waste time at the supermarket; keep a datebook so you don't forget appointments and can schedule them with enough time to arrive without rushing. If you're working on a deadline, block out chunks of time during which you make no appointments and won't let yourself be disturbed. Have designated shelves or drawers for items like keys, household supplies, and important papers, so you don't waste time in a frantic search.

In addition, reexamine your priorities. Does it really matter if you pick up the dry cleaning today or tomorrow? If it does matter, is there another task you can put off instead? Or delegate responsibilities: ask your husband to get the dry cleaning. Hire people to do chores such as cleaning the house or the car. You can't put a price on the relief you'll feel when you lighten your load.

EXERCISE

Virtually every expert on stress reduction extols the benefits of physical exercise. Regular exercise increases your stamina, so your body is less prone to the ravages of stress, and helps you work off the nervous energy you may feel when you're in a fight-or-flight mode. Exercise also helps you relax: it lowers your heart rate and blood pressure and helps you sleep better. Aerobic exercise, such as running or aerobic dance, is particularly good for this purpose because it works out your heart and lungs and helps you burn calories.

You don't have to win the Olympics. No longer are "Go for the burn" and "No pain, no gain" on the lips of exercise advocates. A brisk walk or a relaxing swim can do you just as much good as a three-minute mile—perhaps even more. The most important thing is to find something you can do without undue strain for at least twenty minutes, three times a week. Many people vary their routine—one day they swim, another day they walk, a third day they'll ride a bike—to keep from getting bored.

REGAINING CONTROL

Hundreds of books and thousands of articles have been written on the subject of coping with stress, but the basic message is this: Take control of your life. You can't stop certain things from happening, but you *can* control your response to those events. This chapter has presented some coping techniques designed to help you learn to control those responses, as well as to identify the parts of your life in which you may exert more control than you think. Use these suggestions as a springboard for developing some healthy coping techniques of your own.

SEVEN

LIVING WITH IBS

You *can* live, and live well, with IBS. In fact, you can play a major role in preventing flare-ups, and in seeing to it that the flare-ups that do occur are mild.

In this book you've learned what IBS is—and what it isn't. You've also learned about the various strategies doctors and patients use for managing the symptoms of IBS: diet, drugs, and stress-coping techniques. Every IBS patient is unique, so what works for you may not work for anyone else. If one approach doesn't help, keep trying others—with your doctor's approval—until you hit upon something that works for you.

IBS is your body's way of asking you to slow down and review your life-style. Maybe you have to reorder your priorities, evaluate your eating habits, exercise more, learn how to cope with stress—or perhaps a little of all of these. Whatever you try, be patient. Don't expect miracles overnight, and don't blame yourself if something doesn't work. The very act of taking control of their lives is, for many people, a major relief of stress.

In addition to the forms of treatment already discussed, there are a few more measures that don't fall neatly into any category. Some IBS patients have been helped by one or more of these, others have not. They are presented here for you to consider if you want to leave no stone unturned.

Psychotherapy

When properly conducted, psychotherapy helps reacquaint you with feelings that may have been long buried or repressed, and shows you how those subconscious feelings influence your behavior today. The success of this process depends on your relationship with the therapist, your level of comfort in talking about your feelings, the therapist's technique and personality, the frequency with which you go for treatment, and many other subtle factors. Indeed, psychotherapy is not a cure-all, and its effectiveness in managing IBS is highly debatable. Nevertheless, you may find it helpful for developing new coping skills and putting your problems in perspective.

Support Groups

Several attempts have been made at group therapy for people with IBS, with mixed success. Basically, the groups' goals have been to help the participants get in touch with their feelings, recognize the relationship between tension and IBS, and enhance their skills in coping with stress and communicating.

More research needs to be done on the efficacy of IBS support groups and the best way to conduct them, but it might help just to know you're not alone. Group members can give each other emotional support and offer suggestions for coping with symptoms. For more information about a group in your area, contact the American Digestive Disease Society, whose phone number and address are listed in this chapter.

LIVING WITH IBS—YOU CAN DO IT!

Stress and chronic disease have been the subjects of hundreds of self-help books and workshops, but the advice they offer is easily distilled. They urge you to acknowledge the nature of your problem and the importance of changing your behavior and patterns of thought. They also point out the futility of trying to control others and the importance of keeping the focus on yourself. While all of this is far more easily said than done, those who try it usually find that their lives change for the better, sometimes dramatically, sometimes in more subtle ways. Self-help groups and psychotherapy often help people make these changes, while family therapy may help those who experience problems with family members.

It's important to remember that IBS is a multifaceted condition that may be exacerbated by any number of things. Most of these factors are controllable. Achieving this control takes time, patience, and courage, but you can do it. Ask your doctor before trying something new, don't push yourself too hard, and take things one day at a time. By using the knowledge offered in this book, and getting whatever additional support you need, you may join the millions of IBS sufferers who have learned to control their symptoms and enjoy happy, fulfilling lives.

FOR MORE INFORMATION

Here are the addresses and phone numbers of the organizations mentioned in this book, as well as other organizations that may be able to provide you with more information.

American Celiac Society
45 Gifford Avenue
Jersey City, NJ 07304
(201) 435-2400
Provides assistance to individuals who are allergic to wheat.

American Dietetic Association
216 West Jackson Boulevard
Suite 800
Chicago, IL 60606-6995
(800) 877-1600

American Digestive Disease Society (ADDS)
7720 Wisconsin Avenue
Bethesda, MD 20814
(301) 697-5600

Biofeedback Society of America
10200 W. 44th Avenue, Suite 304
Wheat Ridge, CO 80033
(303) 422-8436
Send a stamped, self-addressed envelope for more information and a list of referrals.

Center for Digestive Disorders
Central DuPage Hospital
25 North Winfield Road
Winfield, IL 60190
(708) 682-1600 ext. 6493

Contact: Diane Minutillo
A multifaceted program for people who suffer from gastro-
    intestinal disorders.

Digestive Disease National Coalition
511 Capitol Court, NE, Suite 300
Washington, DC 20002
(202) 544-7497
This organization informs the public and health care
    professionals about digestive diseases and related
    nutrition.

Ileitis and Colitis Education Foundation
    (see Center for Digestive Disorders)
    Contact: Julie Geiersbach

National Digestive Diseases Information Clearinghouse
Box NDDIC 9000 Rockville Pike
Bethesda, MD 20892
(301) 468-6344

National Foundation for Ileitis and Colitis
444 Park Avenue South
New York, NY 10016
(212) 685-3440

GLOSSARY OF TERMS

acute—An adjective used to describe a medical condition of short duration.

anticholinergic—A drug that inhibits the action of cholinergic nerves, so called because they secrete a chemical known as acetylcholine. These nerves help regulate gut movement, so by suppressing this activity, anticholinergic drugs relieve intestinal cramps.

antidepressant—A drug used in the treatment of clinical depression.

antispasmodic—A drug that decreases the intensity of muscle contractions, or spasms, in the digestive tract.

barium enema—An enema administered for the purpose of X-raying the colon. Barium is a contrast medium that makes the colon visible to the X-ray machine.

cholesystokinin (CCK)—A hormone secreted by the small intestine that stimulates contractions of the digestive tract and influences the action of the gall bladder. CCK is believed to play a role, as yet undefined, in the gut motility problems that occur with IBS.

chronic—A condition of long duration. To make a diagnosis of IBS, some doctors believe symptoms must persist for two years or more.

chronic colitis—Another name for IBS. The name is misleading because IBS actually has nothing to do with colitis.

colon—The final five to six feet of the digestive tract. By the time a meal reaches the colon, all that is left is fluid and waste. Under normal circumstances the colon absorbs much of the fluid to make a solid stool. Also called the large intestine.

colonic neurosis—Another name for irritable bowel syndrome.

colonoscope—A diagnostic instrument consisting of a hollow tube with a light at one end, which enables a doctor to see directly into the colon.

constipation—A hard bowel movement passed with discomfort, difficulty, or pain. Most experts think at least three days must elapse between bowel movements before a patient is truly constipated, but each individual's personal pattern must be taken into account.

Crohn's disease—A chronic, inflammatory disease of the digestive tract that may permanently damage the affected portion of the GI tract, leading to ulceration, malnutrition, intestinal obstruction, and, in serious cases, the formation of fistulas. Also called regional ileitis.

diarrhea—An excessively watery stool, passed with urgency, usually resulting when material passes through the colon too quickly.

diverticulitis—Inflammation of diverticuli (see below).

diverticulosis—The condition in which outpouchings (diverticuli) form in the wall of the digestive tract.

diverticulum—An outpouching that forms in the wall of the digestive tract. Plural form: diverticuli.

endoscopy—The use of an endoscope, a hollow tube with a light attached, to see into an organ. Colonoscopy and sigmoidoscopy are forms of endoscopy.

esophagus—The tube between the throat (pharynx) and the stomach.

fiber—The indigestible part of plant foods such as fruits, vegetables, and grains. Among other things, fiber promotes regularity and keeps the muscles of the digestive tract in good working condition, and may play an important role in the management of IBS.

fistula—An abnormal connection or canal that forms between an inflamed organ and another organ or the skin.

flatulence—The condition of having or passing excessive gas.

functional bowel disease—Another name for irritable bowel syndrome.

functional gastrointestinal disorder—Any condition in which the GI tract does not work the way it is supposed to, even though X rays and other diagnostic methods reveal no sign of disease. Irritable bowel syndrome is a functional gastrointestinal disorder.

gastritis—Inflammation of the stomach that may result from food poisoning or from a long-term condition such as alcoholism.

gastrocolic reflex—The reflexive contraction of the colon in response to food entering the stomach. Some scientists believe IBS symptoms may result, in part, from an exaggerated gastrocolic reflex.

gastroenterologist—A physician who specializes in the treatment of diseases of the digestive tract.

gut—Another name for the digestive tract.

hormone—A chemical released by a gland in one part of the body that works on another part of the body. CCK, for example, is released by the small intestine and works on the gall bladder.

irritable bowel syndrome (IBS)—A functional bowel disorder characterized by excessive motility of the GI tract, particularly the colon. Symptoms of IBS include gas, cramps, bloating, constipation, diarrhea, and alternating episodes of constipation and diarrhea.

irritable colon—Another name for irritable bowel syndrome.

lactose—The sugar that occurs naturally in milk.

lactose intolerance—The inability to digest lactose due to the lack of an intestinal enzyme. The symptoms of lactose intolerance include gas, diarrhea, and cramps.

large intestine—Another name for the colon.

motility—Contractions of the muscle of the digestive tract and movement of its contents.

mucous colitis—Another name for irritable bowel syndrome. This name is misleading because IBS actually has nothing to do with colitis.

nervous stomach, nervous diarrhea—Other terms for irritable bowel syndrome.

placebo—An inactive compound given to a patient who believes the compound has some medicinal effect. Patients frequently improve when taking placebos, a phenomenon physicians call the "placebo effect," which demonstrates the power of suggestion in medical care.

sigmoidoscope—A flexible hollow tube with a light at one end, designed for seeing into the colon. Also see **colonoscope, endoscopy**.

sign—A feature of a patient's condition that the doctor finds during an examination, as opposed to a symptom, which the patient detects himself.

small intestine—The portion of the digestive tract that lies between the stomach and the large intestine. This is where most digestion and virtually all absorption of nutrients into the body occurs.

spasm—A strong and abrupt contraction of a muscle, usually associated with pain. Muscle spasms may last from a few minutes to several hours. Some of the symptoms of IBS are associated with spasms of muscles of the GI tract.

spastic colon, spastic colon syndrome—Other terms for irritable bowel syndrome.

stress—The tensions and strains of daily life which require major life changes or more subtle coping abilities.

Without healthy means of relieving or reducing stress, an individual's health may suffer.

symptom—A characteristic of a condition that the patient detects himself, as opposed to a sign, which the doctor finds during an examination. For example, pain felt by the patient is a symptom, while abdominal tenderness detected by a doctor feeling a patient's stomach is a sign.

ulcerative colitis—A form of chronic colitis characterized by pain, weight loss, ulcerations in the colon, and bloody diarrhea. Ulcerative colitis is curable through surgical removal of the affected portion of the colon.

BIBLIOGRAPHY

Titles prefaced by an asterisk (*) are recommended for further reading.

American Digestive Disease Society. *ADDS Dietary Plans.* Bethesda, Md: ADDs, 1984.

Anker, Vincent. *What to Know About the Treatment of Cancer.* Seattle: Madrona Publishers, 1984.

Berkow, Robert M., and Andrew J. Fletcher, eds. *The Merck Manual of Diagnosis and Therapy.* Volume I: General Medicine. 15th edition. Rahway, N.J.: Merck Sharp & Dohme Research Laboratories, 1987.

Bongiovanni, Gail L., ed. *Essentials of Clinical Gastroenterology.* New York: McGraw-Hill, Inc., 1988.

*Danzi, J. Thomas. *Free Yourself From Digestive Pain.* Englewood Cliffs, N.J.: Prentice-Hall, Inc. 1984.

Davenport, Horace W. *A Digest of Digestion.* Chicago: Year Book Medical Publishers, Inc., 1973.

Dodge, David L., and Walter T. Martin. *Social Stress and Chronic Illness.* Notre Dame, Ind: University of Notre Dame Press, 1970.

Dorland's Illustrated Medical Dictionary, 27th edition. Philadelphia: W.B. Saunders Co., 1988.

Gibbons, Thomas B. *How Doctors Diagnose You and How You Can Help*. Philadelphia: The Saunders Press, 1980.

*Glucksberg, Harold, and Jack W. Singer. *Cancer Care: A Personal Guide*. New York: Charles Scribner's Sons, 1982.

*Goldberg, Myron D., and Julie Rubin. *The Inside Tract: Understanding and Preventing Digestive Disorders*. Washington, D.C.: The American Association of Retired Persons, 1986.

Jamowitz, Henry D. *Your Gut Feelings: A Complete Guide to Living Better with Intestinal Problems*. New York: Oxford University Press, 1987.

Langman, M.J.S.: *A Concise Textbook of Gastroenterology*. Second Edition. Edinburgh, Scotland: Churchill Livingstone, 1982.

Levitt, Paul M., and Elissa Guralnick, with Dr. A. Robert Kagan and Dr. Harvey Gilbert. *The Cancer Reference Book*. New York: Facts on File, Inc., 1983.

Long, James W. *The Essential Guide to Prescription Drugs—1989*. New York: Harper & Row Publishers, Inc., 1989.

McKhann, Charles F. *The Facts About Cancer*. Englewood Cliffs, N.J.: Prentice-Hall, Inc., 1981.

Napoli, Maryann. *Health Facts: A Critical Evaluation of the Major Problems, Treatments, and Alternatives Facing Medical Consumers*. Woodstock, N.Y.: Overlook Press, 1982.

*Plaut, Martin E. *The Doctor's Guide to You and Your Colon*. New York: Harper & Row Publishers, Inc., 1982.

*Shaffer, Martin. *Life After Stress*. Chicago: Contemporary Books, 1983.

*Shimberg, Elaine Fantle. *Relief From IBS.* New York: M. Evans & Company, Inc., 1988.

U.S. Pharmacopeial Convention, Inc. *Drug Information for the Consumer.* Mount Vernon, N.Y.: Consumers Union, 1987.

Whitney, Eleanor Noss, and Eva May Nunnelley Hamilton. *Understanding Nutrition.* St. Paul, Minn.: West Publishing Co., 1981.

ABOUT THE AUTHOR

Norra Tannenhaus holds degrees in biopsychology and nutrition from Vassar College and Columbia University. She has written extensively on health, medicine, and nutrition for consumers and physicians, and her magazine articles have appeared in such major publications as *Self, Glamour,* and *Mademoiselle. Learning to Live with Chronic IBS* is her fourth book. Although she is a New Yorker at heart, Ms. Tannenhaus currently makes her home in Los Angeles.